Martial Arts Instruction for Children

Special Concerns for Teachers and Parents

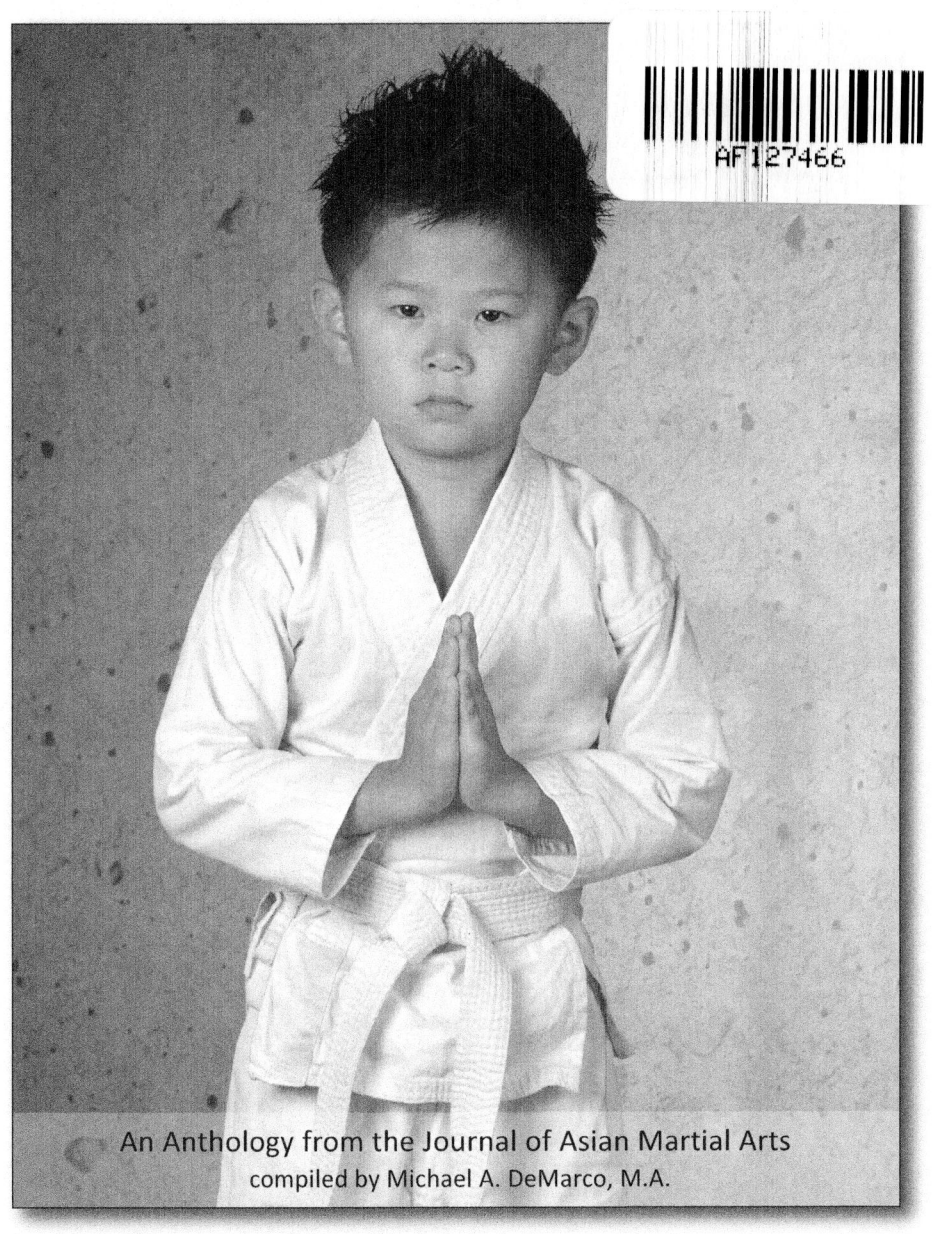

An Anthology from the Journal of Asian Martial Arts
compiled by Michael A. DeMarco, M.A.

Disclaimer
Please note that the authors and publisher of this book are not responsible in any manner whatsoever for any injury that may result from practicing the techniques and/or following the instructions given within. Since the physical activities described herein may be too strenuous in nature for some readers to engage in safely, it is essential that a physician be consulted prior to training.

All Rights Reserved
No part of this publication, including illustrations, may be reproduced or utilized in any form or by any means, electronic or mechanical, including photocopying, recording, or by any information storage and retrieval system (beyond that copying permitted by sections 107 and 108 of the US Copyright Law and except by reviewers for the public press), without written permission from Via Media Publishing Company.

Warning: Any unauthorized act in relation to a copyright work may result in both a civil claim for damages and criminal prosecution.

Copyright © 2020
by Via Media Publishing Company

Articles in this anthology were originally published in the *Journal of Asian Martial Arts*. Listed according to the table of contents for this anthology:

Boudreau, F., et al. (1995), Vol. 4 No. 4, pp. 50–69
Hendrey, E. (1997), Vol. 6 No. 2, pp. 80-95
Yoshinaga, S. (2000), Vol. 9 No. 2, pp. 80–89
Webster-Doyle, T. (2003), Vol. 12 No. 1, pp. 88–89
Barnfield, A. (2003), Vol. 12 No. 3, pp. 8–17
Cooper, E. (2006), Vol. 15 No. 4, pp. 20–29
Van Rheenan, D. (2011), Vol. 20 No. 4, pp. 8–25
Paul, J. (2009), Vol. 20 No. 4, pp. 36–51

Cover Illustrations
Photograph and copyright by olegdudko.
Image ID: 46794972 courtesy of 123RF.com

Print Edition
ISBN-13: 9798568446767

www.viamediapublishing.com

contents

iv   Preface
       by Michael DeMarco, M.A.

CHAPTERS

1   Psychological and Physical Changes in School-Age Karate Participants: Parental Observations
      by Françoise Boudreau, Ph.D., Ralph Folman, M.D., and Burt Konzak, Ph.D.

21   Viewing Human Conflict Through the Martial Arts: Interview with Dr. Terrance Webster-Doyle
       by Elisa Hendrey, M.A.

39   Kon and Haku: The Spirit of Heaven and Earth in Children
       by Sakuyama Yoshinaga, B.A., translated by Duncan Robert Mark

47   Educating the Mind as Well as the Body Through Martial Arts Training
       by Terrence Webster-Doyle, Ph.D.

51   Observational Learning in the Martial Art Studio: Instructors as Models of Positive Behaviors
       by Anne M.C. Barnfield, Ph.D.

65   Information and Strategies for Martial Arts Instructors Working with Children Diagnosed with Attention-Deficit/Hyperactivity Disorder
       by Eric K. Cooper, Ph.D.

79   Reflections on an After-School Literacy Program and the Educational Value of Taekwondo: A Preliminary Analysis
       by Derek Van Rheenen, Ph.D.

99   Teaching Aikido to Children with Autism Spectrum Disorders
       by Josh Paul, M.A.

115   Index

preface

This anthology isn't a typical "How To" book for teaching martial arts to children. The eight chapters included tend not only to the physical aspects of the instruction of skills, but give special attention to the essential nature of children, their body and minds, and the effects their train have on socialization. In addition, some authors write specifically on the special needs of children with autism, attention deficit, and hyperactivity disorders.

As young children learn about the world over time, what activities they do influence their outlooks and influence their behaviors. Will enrolled into a martial arts class make them aggressive and perhaps violent? Or, will they learn how to have self-control and obtain skills that bring about conflict resolution?

Many martial arts instructors are highly skilled in self-defense. As Dr. Webster-Doyle shows, martial arts instruction should also nurture the students' minds to be responsible for what they are learning. Unfortunately, many instructors may not be so prepared for providing a balance for teaching the physical as well as the mental aspects. Dr. Barnfield's chapter is clear on how instructors are models of behavior.

The chapter by Dr. Van Rheenan illustrates how traditional marital arts instruction can benefit children in way outside the dojo. What they learn in the studio—discipline, respect, effort, etc.—can be applied to ways of behavior at home and at school.

Two chapters focus on children with special needs. Dr. Cooper's writing looks closely at attention-deficit and hyperactivity disorders. He clarifies just what these disorders entail so instructors can better understand their students and proved the best possible instruction. Josh Paul's chapter is similar, but focuses on Autism Spectrum Disorders and includes a technical section of Aikido-based practices for the dojo.

Parents and instructors will benefit from the content provided in this special anthology since it focuses on children as students of martial arts. The former will see the potential a martial arts school can offer to their children. The later will find ways to improve their instruction.

Michael A. DeMarco, Publisher
Santa Fe, New Mexico, December 2020

chapter 1

Psychological and Physical Changes in School-Age Karate Participants: Parental Observations

by Françoise Boudreau, Ph.D., Ralph Folman, M.D., and Burt Konzak, Ph.D.

*This study was funded by the Social Sciences and Humanities Research Council.

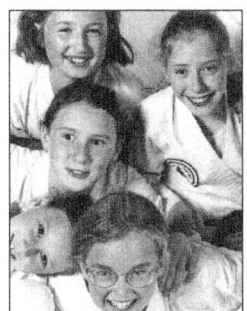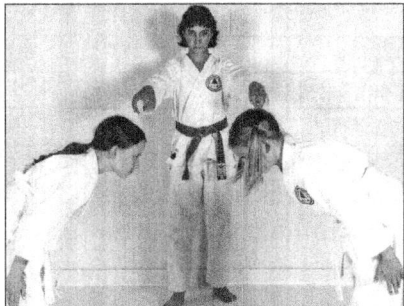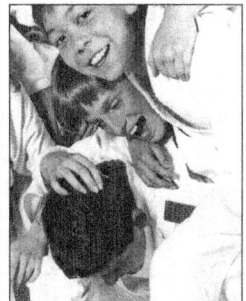

Photography courtesy of Donna Maloney.

Traditional karate-do is an Eastern martial art that in its pure form incorporates physical and mental (psychological) training. The authors, as teachers and practitioners of karate, have noted its beneficial effects on the behavior and physical well-being of school-aged children. To test these observations, questionnaires were distributed to the parents of school-aged participants enrolled in a traditional karate program in order to ascertain the perceived benefits of the training on the children. Responses were obtained from parents of 102 beginners and 72 non-beginners. The data were analyzed both by rank (i.e., advancement in the training) and gender. Parents perceived a large increase in "self-confidence," "self-worth" or "self-esteem" as the single most obvious benefit attributable to the karate training. This benefit was more pronounced as the trainee advanced in ranking, and girls were reported to show a much higher increase in self-confidence than boys. Benefits in the area of physical health were also noted.

Self-confidence and self-esteem are generally accepted as fundamental to the healthy emotional and mental development of children (Levine and Satz, 1984; Corbin and Nix, 1979). Attainment of good physical coordination and ability is obviously desirable as well and has been documented to affect self-esteem (Miller, 1989; Shaw, et. al., 1982) mental development, and academic performance (Shephard, 1982; Sinclair, 1983). In North American culture, for example, athletic prowess is held in high regard, both in schools and in society at large, even though most people are merely spectators.

Despite the positive effect of physical activity on the development of self-esteem, numerous studies (Hansen and McKenzie, 1988; Croce and Lavay, 1987) have documented that North American children do not participate nearly enough, either as individuals or in organized school programs. This deficiency has been aggravated by the failure of most secondary school and university and college authorities to require compulsory enrollment of their students in physical education programs (Hansen and McKenzie, 1988; Taylor, 1986), even though the post-pubertal individual needs regular exercise the most (Grace, 1987).

Karate-do, "empty hand method," is a martial art with a history and tradition dating back centuries to ancient Buddhism, particularly in China and Japan. In its traditional form, it emphasizes self-development, both physical and mental, and rewards individual growth rather than victory over others. As practiced today, there is no preselection of participants, whether by age, sex, size, or athletic aptitude. It is both physically and mentally rigorous. Karate training has always used methods that seek to increase proprioceptive awareness and thereby enhance balance, coordination, and power. (In this report, the term *karate-do* is used in its traditional sense, as opposed to some of the modern altered forms, such as kick-boxing or full-contact karate, which neglect the mental and philosophical components considered so essential in the traditional art, emphasizing instead its potentially violent aspects.)

While teaching and participating in a school of traditional karate, the authors noted that the training appeared to exert a highly beneficial effect on the behavior and physical well-being of participating school-aged children. Anecdotal reports provided by staff of the Child Development Clinic, The Hospital for Sick Children (W. Roberts, personal communication, 1991) and by others (Block and Rash, 1981) support our observations. In this exploratory study, we attempted to verify our observations in an objective, quantitative fashion as a preliminary to further, more sophisticated research.

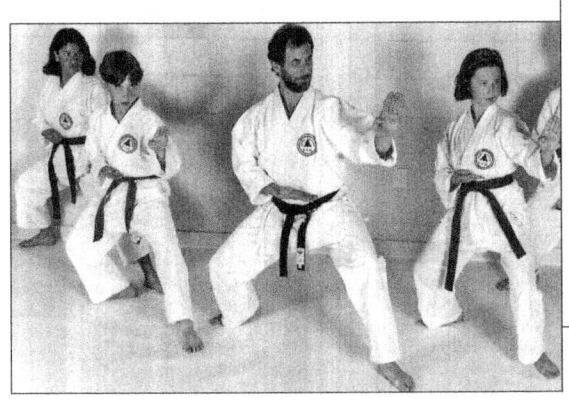
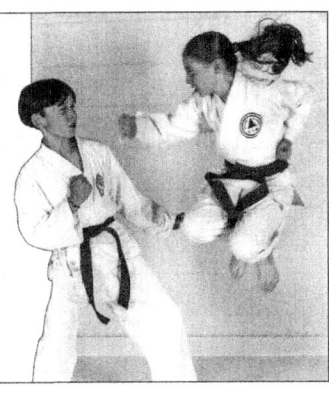

Methods

A questionnaire designed to determine parental expectations of and attitudes toward karate was administered to the parents of 271 children, aged seven to sixteen, who were enrolled in the main Karate School of the Toronto Academy of Karate and six outreach programs taught by advanced-rank student from the main school, located in Toronto, Canada. The children were divided into beginners and non-beginners. The following questions were posed to the parents of the beginners:

1) Would you kindly tell us why you have decided to enroll your child in karate in the first place? Please be as specific as possible.
2) What were your expectations from karate at the time?
3) Do you have any reservations about the karate training?
4) What led you to choose this karate program?

Parents of non-beginners (children who had entered the program before the beginning of the study) were given a questionnaire that included questions 1 and 2 from the beginners' questionnaire, plus the following:

3) Have your expectations of karate changed since you first enrolled your child?
4) What impact do you believe karate training has had on your child since he/she first began? What changes in your child do you attribute mainly to karate training (please be as specific as possible, e.g., improved behavior at home, does better in school, gets into more fights with other kids, has more friends...).

5) In relation to your answer to Question #4, what in your mind is the single most important benefit your child has gained from training?
6) Have you observed any change in your child's "physical health" which you would attribute to the karate training?
- Have visits to the doctor decreased?
- Has he/she had to miss school less often because of illness?
- Does he/she look to you generally more physically healthy?

The questionnaires were distributed in class to the children with instructions to have their parents fill them out and return them at a subsequent class. After all the forms had been collected, the data were analyzed and coded by extracting from the responses a set of appropriate categories of answers to each question. These categories were chosen after all the data had been scrutinized to judge the range of possible answers to each question. Thus, for Question 1, "Why have you decided to enroll your child in karate?" the following six categories were identified:

a) for physical improvement
b) for improvement in mental skills and relations, subdivided into: (i) self-discipline; (ii) self-confidence; (iii) other
c) for academic improvement
d) child asked to join
e) for development of self-defense skills
f) other.

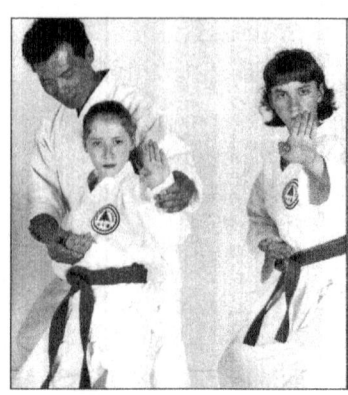

A similar process was carried out for the rest of the questions. All the data were analyzed by one codifier, who carried out internal validity checks by randomly returning several times to the data and recoding the answers to see if the same categories emerged. This was almost always the case.

The results were divided into two broad groupings, "Beginners" and "Non-Beginners." The scores per category for each group were summed and the percentages of the totals calculated (Tables 1-3, Graph 1). The percentages were then used to calculate "Difference Scores," which were graphed to show the relative importance of specific categories for different sets of parents (Graphs 2-3). An open bar on a Difference Score graph indicates more importance for parents of girls; a solid bar, more importance for parents of boys; and a neutral (or zero) value, equal importance to both sets of parents.

The information given by one non-beginner girl was excluded because she appeared to have filled out the parents' questionnaire herself, and that of one non-beginner boy was only partially useable because his belt-ranking was not specified. The belt ranks used are white (beginner), yellow, green, blue, purple, brown, and black. (These ranks and colors may vary among karate schools.)

The analysis by gender was complicated by the fact that there were fourteen non-beginner boys in the white rank but no corresponding group of girls. We, therefore, analyzed the data of the two corresponding groups (i.e., girls in the yellow rank and above versus boys in the yellow rank and above) and compared the findings to the results for all the non-beginner boys versus all non-beginner girls. The results differed in minor ways only. However, to keep the comparison as valid as possible, we chose for discussion the two corresponding groups, excluding the fourteen boys in the white rank from our results.

Results

In total, 102 parental responses were received in the beginner category and 72 in the non-beginner. These were analyzed by gender for the beginners, and by belt-ranking as well as gender for non-beginners.

Beginners (85 Boys, 17 Girls)

The reasons for enrollment (Question 1) given by parents of beginners included all categories from "improvement in mental skills and relations" to "other" (Table 1, Graph 1). Answers related to psychological improvement included "self-discipline," "self-confidence," and other factors in psychological well-being. The "other" category included such reasons as "for the child to have fun," "for something different to do," or "to learn the basic techniques and philosophy of karate." Parents often gave several reasons.

The most common answers to Question 2, on expectations, were the same as for Question 1 because of the similarity of the two questions (Table 1). Other answers included "to learn the serious side of karate—that it isn't a game," "to get true appreciation of karate—not the TV version," "control over her life," and "break out of helpless mold."

In response to Question 3, 46.1% of parents had some reservations about the training; these were mainly that the child would be hurt (7.8%) or hurt others (25.5%). Parents of boys expressed the fear that their child would hurt others, much more than did parents of girls (Table 1, Graph 2).

Analysis by sex showed more striking results, some of them unexpected (Table 1, Graph 2). Parents of girls had quite different expectations of karate than those of boys. Girls' parents enrolled their children chiefly to help them obtain psychological and physical benefits and to acquire self-defense skills, whereas the chief reason boys were enrolled was that they asked to join. In response to Question 4, "convenience" of the program was a chief reason why boys were enrolled, whereas "university affiliation" and "quality of the program and the instructors" were prime reasons given by the parents of girls. (For most of the participating children, the time commitment demanded by karate, and by this program in particular, precluded involvement in any additional extracurricular sport.)

Non-Beginners (64 Boys, 8 Girls)

Data on non-beginners were analyzed by gender (Table 2 and Graph 3) and by belt-ranking (white-yellow, green-blue, purple-brown) (Table 3 and Graph 1).

Although enrollment reasons and expectations were roughly similar to those provided by beginners, some categories of answers to Questions 1-3 did change dramatically. For example, psychological improvement was cited as an enrollment reason by 64.0% of parents of male non-beginners in contrast to 41.2% of parents of beginners. It may be that the perceived changes in non-beginner boys modified parents' memories of their original enrollment reasons. The great majority of parents indicated no changes in expectations since their child had been enrolled in the program.

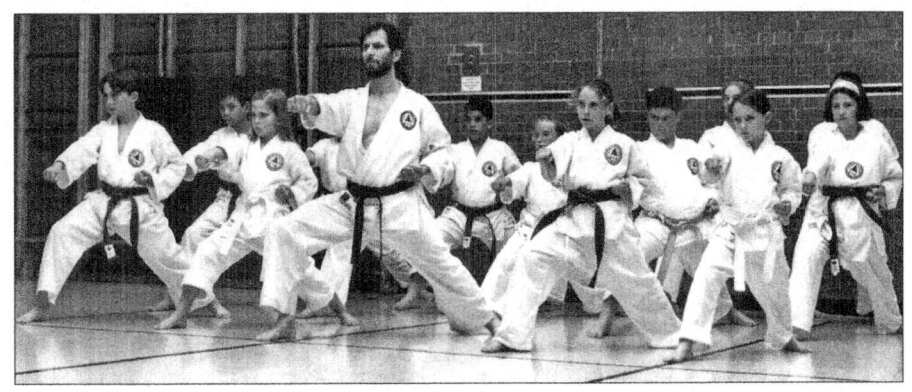

The most dramatic improvement (Question 4) was reported by parents of girls (Table 2, Graph 3), 100% of whom noted an increase in self-confidence (vs. 58% of boys). Increase in self-discipline was reported by 50% of girls' parents vs. 30% of boys' parents. Physical improvements were noted in 50% of girls vs. 36% of boys and academic improvement in 37.5% of girls vs. 14% of boys. "Other" changes were noted in 62.5% of girls (vs. 32.0% in boys). Examples included "awareness of her potential and abilities," "commitment," and "competing with self instead of others." In the boys, "other" benefits, reported by 32% of parents, included "realizes everyone starts from bottom," "listens better," and "learning lessons of tremendous benefit throughout life." Many parents of boys gave extensive multiple answers.

The single most pervasive benefit attributed to karate (Question 5), observed across both sexes and belt-rankings, were parental perceptions of an increase in "self-confidence," "self-worth," or "self-esteem." This benefit became more pronounced with advances in belt-ranking, being reported by 83.3% of the parents of children in the purple-brown ranks, 61.1% in the green-blue ranks, and 47.6% in the white-yellow ranks. In response to Question 4, on changes attributable to karate, the only parents reporting "no difference yet" were those of the white-yellow (19.0%) and green-blue belts (5.6%). All parents of children in the more advanced rankings (purple-brown belts) noted definite changes: None of them reported "no difference yet," and 91.7% noted "increase in self-confidence" as an important change versus 61.1 % for the green-blue belt group and 45.2% for the white-yellow belt group.

In response to Question 6 on changes in physical health (admittedly a leading question), 26.1% of the parents of white-yellow belts noted general physical benefits, 28.6% reported fewer visits to the doctor and 14.3% less school missed, and 47.6% agreed that their child looked healthier. A marked increase in these percentages was reported for the higher belt rankings: 55.6% of the green-blue belts reported beneficial changes in general physical health and felt that their child "looked healthier," 33.3% noted fewer doctor visits, and 22.2% reported less school missed. These percentages were even higher for children in the purple-brown category.

The relationships between the answers from the boys' parents and those of the girls' parents are illustrated in the "difference-score" graphs.

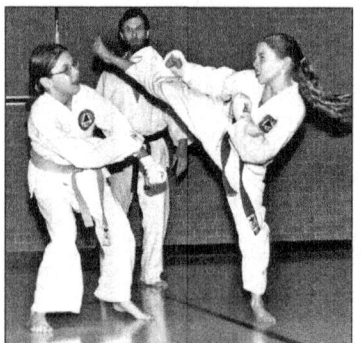
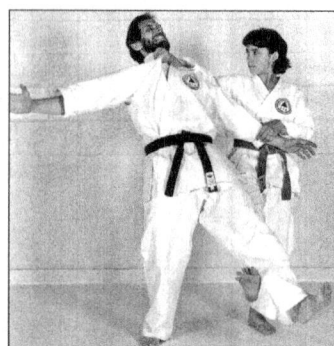
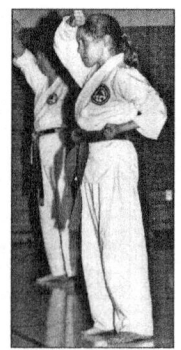
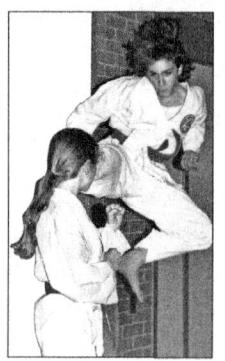
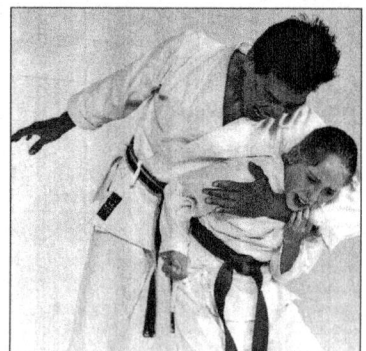
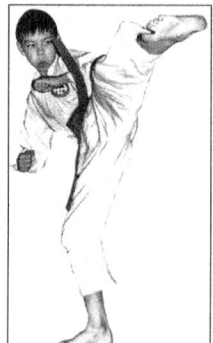

Discussion

Discussion of the results can be divided into two main categories: physical and psychological.

On the physical level, the parents of the participants reported definite benefits as a result of the activity, from "looking healthier" to less school absenteeism and less need for visits to doctors. These benefits increased in proportion to the length of time in the karate program and the achievement of more advanced ranking. The beneficial impact of regular exercise on physical health has been documented recently by studies in France and Canada (Hansen and McKenzie, 1988; Grace, 1987).

The benefits of regular physical activity for intellectual and academic performance have also been documented, although not as decisively, in the Trois Rivieres and Vanves studies (Shepard, 1982). One of these studies (Trois Rivieres) showed that girls from a rural school benefitted most, an interesting finding in the light of our results showing how much benefit girls derived from the program. A thorough review of the effects of physical activity on intellectual and academic performance was undertaken by Kirkendall (1985). He concluded that there is a moderate positive relationship between motor performance and intellectual performance, especially with coordination and balance tasks, but that this entire area of study needs further research.

In general, most parents reported marked increases in their children's self-esteem and self-confidence. While the parents of boys had their expectations fulfilled, often to a greater degree than anticipated, the girls actually surprised their parents—and in a highly positive way. These parents anticipated development of simple self-defense skills and perhaps some increase in self-confidence as a by-product. What they saw was a much greater increase in self-esteem than expected, plus more self-discipline and assertiveness. The parents of boys also noted a marked improvement in interpersonal relations. These findings lead us to speculate that karate-do may permit a resocialization of girls and boys; for example, parents may perceive that it helps fill gaps in our traditional gender socialization, compensating for lack of self-confidence in girls and the lack of sensitivity often perceived among boys.

A similar resocialization process across stereotypical lines was observed in an earlier study with adults (Konzak and Boudreau, 1984), which demonstrated that women black-belts, while remaining as sensitive and tender as) women with lower belt-rankings and women in the general population, were much more self-assured and assertive than other women. Men black-belts had the opposite experience: still assured and assertive, they became more sensitive and gentle than lower-belt men and men in the general population. The result was a "black-belt person" who is at the same time strong and sensitive, powerful and gentle, manifesting the qualities emphasized in the traditional philosophy of karate. Karate-do, it was perceived, liberated the woman in every man \ and the man in every woman. In a preliminary way, the parents' responses suggest that we may be observing a similar process in the children. We are currently involved in a longitudinal study of these children that may provide further evidence for the credibility of this hypothesis.

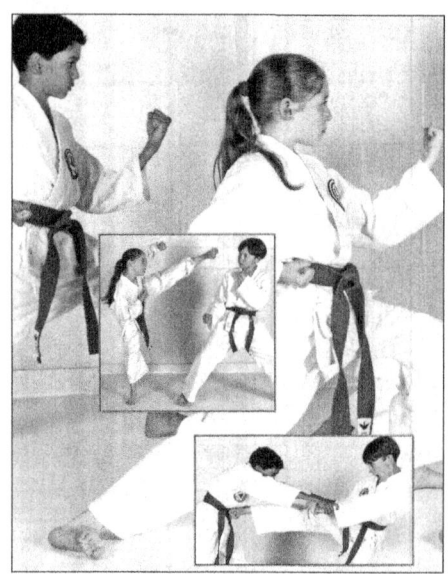 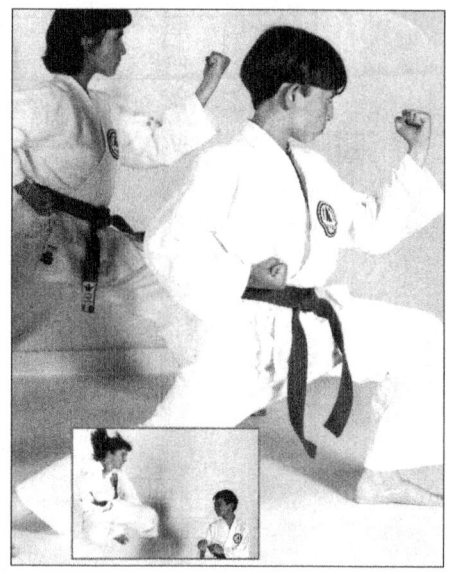

Unfortunately, few girls persist long enough in karate training to obtain its full benefits. Cultural and peer pressures may be responsible; karate training is still not a fashionable activity for female teenagers, and the usual categorization of sports activities into male or female also sets up a barrier (Corbin and Nix, 1979). In addition, karate-do is perceived by the general public as a promoter of aggression. This view has been shown to be fallacious as applied to traditional karate, which has its roots in Zen philosophy and training-hall etiquette that teaches respect for others as well as for self and emphasizes humility while developing self-confidence (Nosanchuk and NacNeil, 1989).

We were impressed by the extensive answers of some parents, who even ascribed "miraculous" benefits to the karate training for their child. Although anecdotal, these parental documents nevertheless convey strong convictions.

A need exists for a sport or physical activity that is open to all, does not require expensive equipment or facilities, does not preselect only the biggest, fastest or tallest, and offers both physical and psychological benefits. Karate-do is such an activity. Our findings provide strong support for the significant mental and physical benefits of traditional karate-do training for young people.

TABLE 1: Responses from Parents of Beginners[a]

QUESTION	Boys (n = 85)	Girls (n = 17)	Total (n = 102)
1) Enrollment reasons			
Physical improvement	31.8	41.2	33.3
Psychological improvement	41.2	64.7	45.1
Self-discipline[b]	30.6	35.3	31.4
Self-confidence	30.6	41.2	32.4
Other	11.8	17.6	12.7
Academic improvement	1.2	5.9	2.0
Child asked to join	45.9	29.4	43.1
Self-defense	22.4	47.1	26.5
Other reasons	35.3	35.3	35.3
2) Enrollment expectations			
Physical improvement	27.1	29.4	27.5
Psychological improvement	56.5	41.2	54.9
Self-discipline[b]	28.2	17.6	26.5
Self-confidence	28.2	41.2	30.4
Other	9.4	11.8	9.8
Academic improvement	1.2	0	1.0
Child asked to join	10.6	23.5	12.7
Self-defense	58.8	58.8	58.8
Other reasons	5.9	0	5.9
3) Reservations about karate			
No	50.6	52.9	51.0
Yes	45.9	47.1	46.1
Child would be hurt	7.1	11.8	7.8
Would hurt others	28.2	11.8	25.5
Both of above	3.5	5.9	3.9
Other[c]	7.1	17.6	8.8
4) Reason for choosing this program			
University affiliation	12.9	41.2	17.6
Quality of the instructors	27.1	52.9	31.4
Private recommendation	12.9	5.9	11.8
Convenient	40.0	35.3	39.2
Other	17.6	1.8	16.8

[a] Responses are expressed as percentages of total in each group.
[b] Subset percentages are also of total in each group.
[c] Too young, overestimate own ability, reluctant, concern about self-defense, asthmatic, too few girls enrolled.

TABLE 2: Responses from Parents of Non-Beginners, by Gender[a]

QUESTION	Boys (n = 50)	Girls (n = 8)
1) Enrollment reasons (Graph 3)		
Physical improvement	46.0	25.0
Psychological improvement	64.0	12.5
Academic improvement	6.0	-
Child asked to join	34.0	12.5
Self-defense	38.0	37.5
Other reasons	36.0	37.5
2) Enrollment expectations (Graph 3)		
Physical improvement	56.0	62.5
Psychological improvement	76.0	37.5
Academic improvement	2.0	-
Self-defense	22.0	37.5
Other expectations	46.0	62.5
3) Changes in expectations (Graph 3)		
No	22.0	37.5
Yes	74.0	62.5
No Response	4.0	-
4) Changes attributable to karate (Graph 3)		
Physical improvement	36.0	50.0
Psychological improvement		
Self-discipline[b]	30.0	50.0
Self-confidence	58.0	100.0
Other	10.0	12.5
Interpersonal relations	42.0	37.5
Academic improvement	14.0	37.5
Other changes	32.0	62.5
No difference yet	10.0	-
No response	2.0	-
5) Single most important benefit (Graph 3)		
Physical improvement	10.0	-
Psychological improvement		
Self-discipline[b]	22.0	37.5
Self-confidence	58.0	87.5
Interpersonal relations	28.0	12.5
Academic	4.0	-
Other benefits	28.0	37.5
No response	6.0	-

[a] Responses are expressed as percentages of total in each group. The column for total percentage (boys/girls) was omitted because of the preponderance of boys in this population.
[b] Subset percentages are also of total in each group.

TABLE 2: continued

QUESTION	Boys (n = 50)	Girls (n = 8)
6) Changes in physical health?		
Yes	42.0	50.0
No	52.0	50.0
No response	6.0	-
Fewer doctor visits		
Yes	36.0	37.5
No	64.0	62.5
Less school missed		
Yes	22.0	37.5
No	78.0	62.5
Looks healthier		
Yes	58.0	87.5
No	42.0	12.5

[a] Responses are expressed as percentages of total in each group.
[b] Subset percentages are also of total in each group.

TABLE 3: Responses from Parents of Non-Beginners, by Ranking[a]

QUESTION	Belt Rankings		
	White & Yellow (n = 42)	Green & Blue (n = 18)	Purple & Brown (n = 12)
1) Enrollment reasons (Graph 1)			
Physical improvement	40.5	61.1	33.3
Psychological improvement	61.9	66.7	58.3
Academic improvement	2.4	-	8.3
Child asked to join	31.0	38.9	25.0
Self-defense	45.2	27.8	41.7
Other reasons	33.3	44.4	16.7
2) Enrollment expectations (Graph 1)			
Physical improvement	61.9	66.7	33.3
Psychological improvement	66.7	77.8	75.0
Academic improvement	7.1	-	-
Self-defense	33.3	16.7	25.0
Other expectations	45.2	50.0	41.7
3) Changes in expectations (Graph 1)			
No	11.9	33.3	41.7
Yes	83.3	66.7	58.3
No Response	4.8	-	-

TABLE 3: Continued

QUESTION	Belt Rankings		
	White & Yellow (n = 42)	Green & Blue (n = 18)	Purple & Brown (n = 12)
4) Changes attributable to karate (Graph 1)			
Physical improvement	28.6	38.9	50.0
Psychological improvement			
Self-discipline[b]	14.3	55.6	33.3
Self-confidence	45.2	61.1	91.7
Sense of responsibility	9.5	11.1	8.3
Interpersonal relations	38.1	50.0	50.0
Academic improvement	7.1	16.7	33.3
Other changes	40.5	38.9	50.0
No difference yet	19.0	5.6	-
No response	2.4	-	-
5) Single most important benefit (Graph 1)			
Physical improvement	11.9	5.6	8.3
Psychological improvement			
Self-discipline[b]	16.7	33.3	25.0
Self-confidence	47.0	61.1	83.3
Interpersonal relations	21.4	27.8	33.4
Academic improvement	-	-	16.7
Other changes	28.6	27.8	25.0
No response	11.9	-	-
6) Changes in physical health (Graph 1)			
Yes	26.1	55.6	75.0
No	69.0	44.4	16.7
No response	4.8	-	8.3
Fewer doctor visits			
Yes	28.6	33.3	66.7
No	71.4	66.7	33.3
Less school missed			
Yes	14.3	33.3	58.3
No	85.7	66.7	41.7
Looks healthier			
Yes	47.6	55.6	100.0
No	52.9	44.4	-

[a] Responses are expressed as percentages of total in each group.
[b] Subset percentages are also of total in each group.

GRAPH 1, PART I: Responses from Parents, by Student Ranking

Questions 1-2 apply to beginners only, and
Questions 1-6 to all non-beginners.

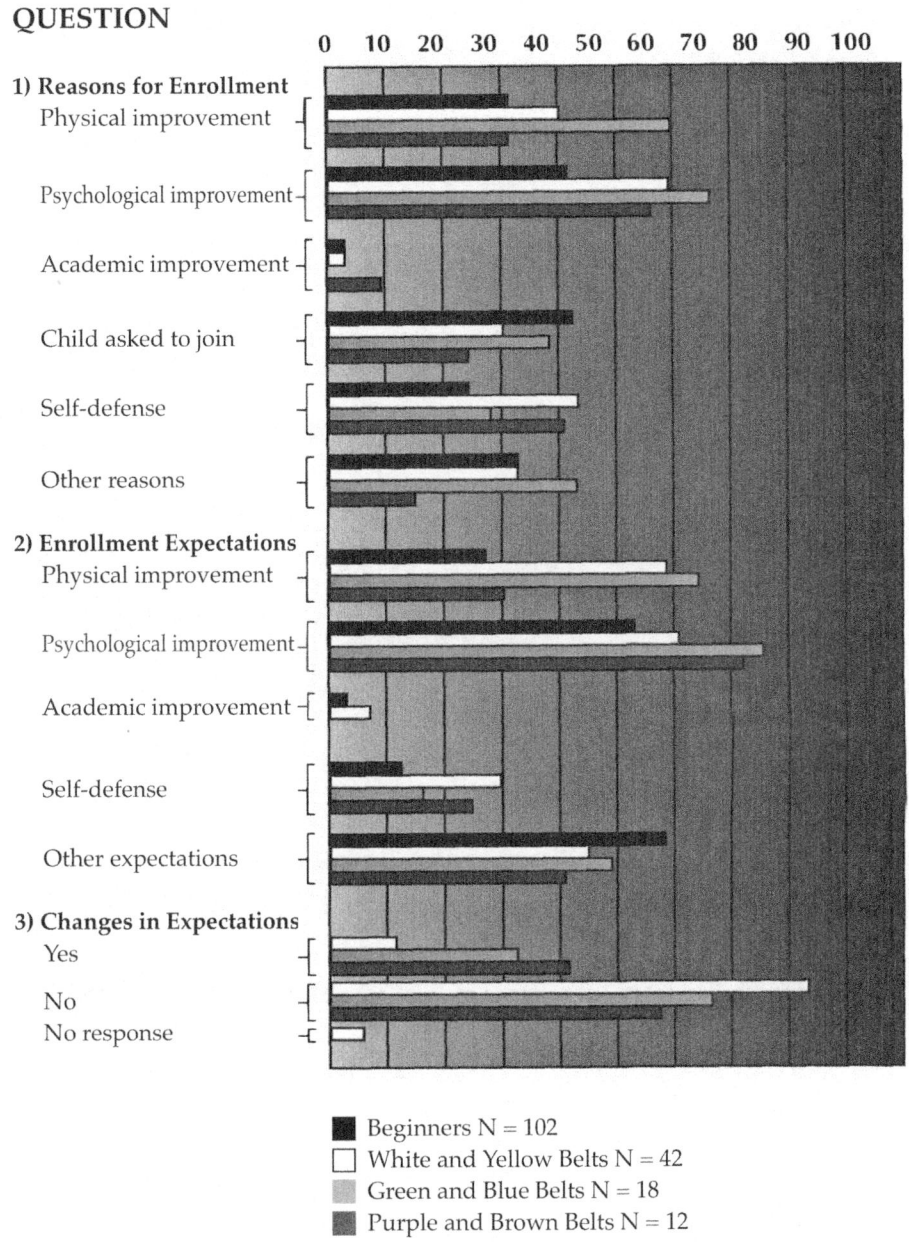

GRAPH 1, PART II

QUESTION

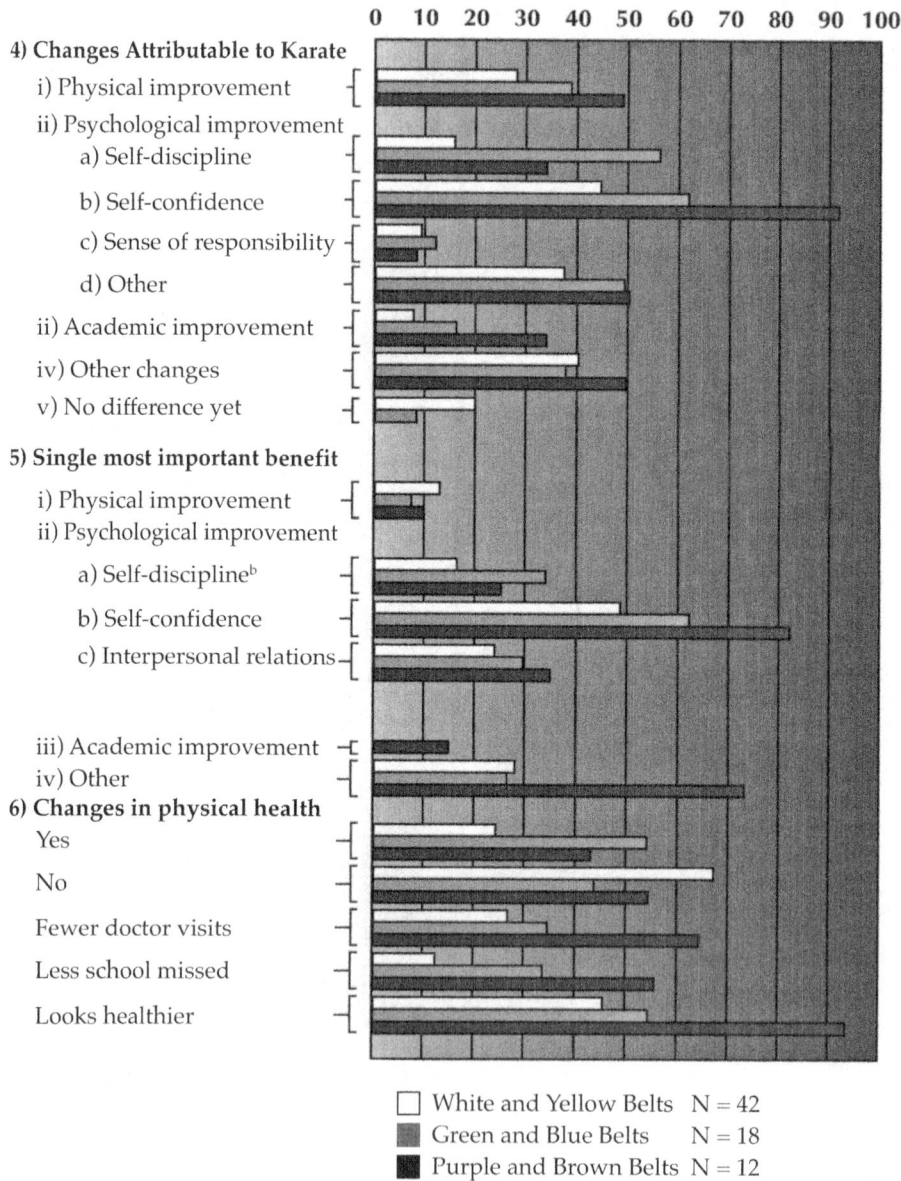

GRAPH 2: Difference Scores Between Boys and Girls Who Were Beginners in the Program

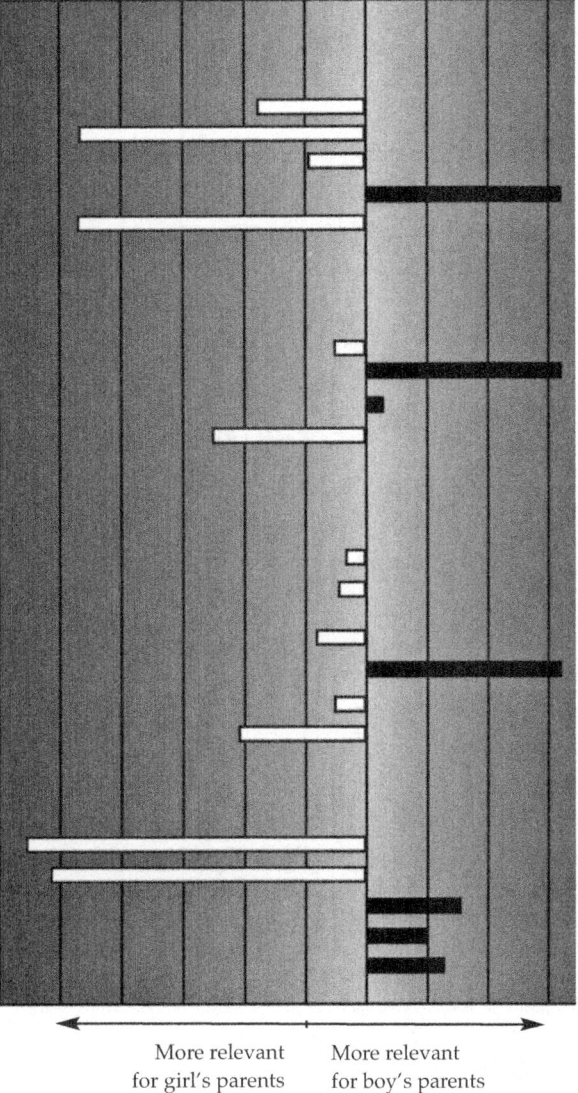

GRAPH 3: Difference Scores between Boys and Girls Who Were Already Enrolled in the Program

1) Reasons for Enrollment

Physical improvement
Psychological improvement
Academic improvement
Child asked to join
Self-defense
Other reasons

2) Enrollment Expectations

Physical improvement
Psychological improvement
Academic improvement
Self-defense
Other reasons

3) Changes in Expectations

Yes
No

4) Changes Attributable to Karate

i) Physical improvement

ii) Psychological improvement
   a) Self-discipline[b]
   b) Self-confidence
   c) Sense of responsibility
   d) Interpersonal relations

iii) Academic improvement

iv) Other

v) No difference yet

5) Most Important Benefit Noted

i) Physical improvement

ii) Psychological improvement
   a) Self-discipline[b]
   b) Self-confidence
   c) Interpersonal relations

iii) Academic improvement

iv) Other

Text for Graph 3 aligns with the following image.

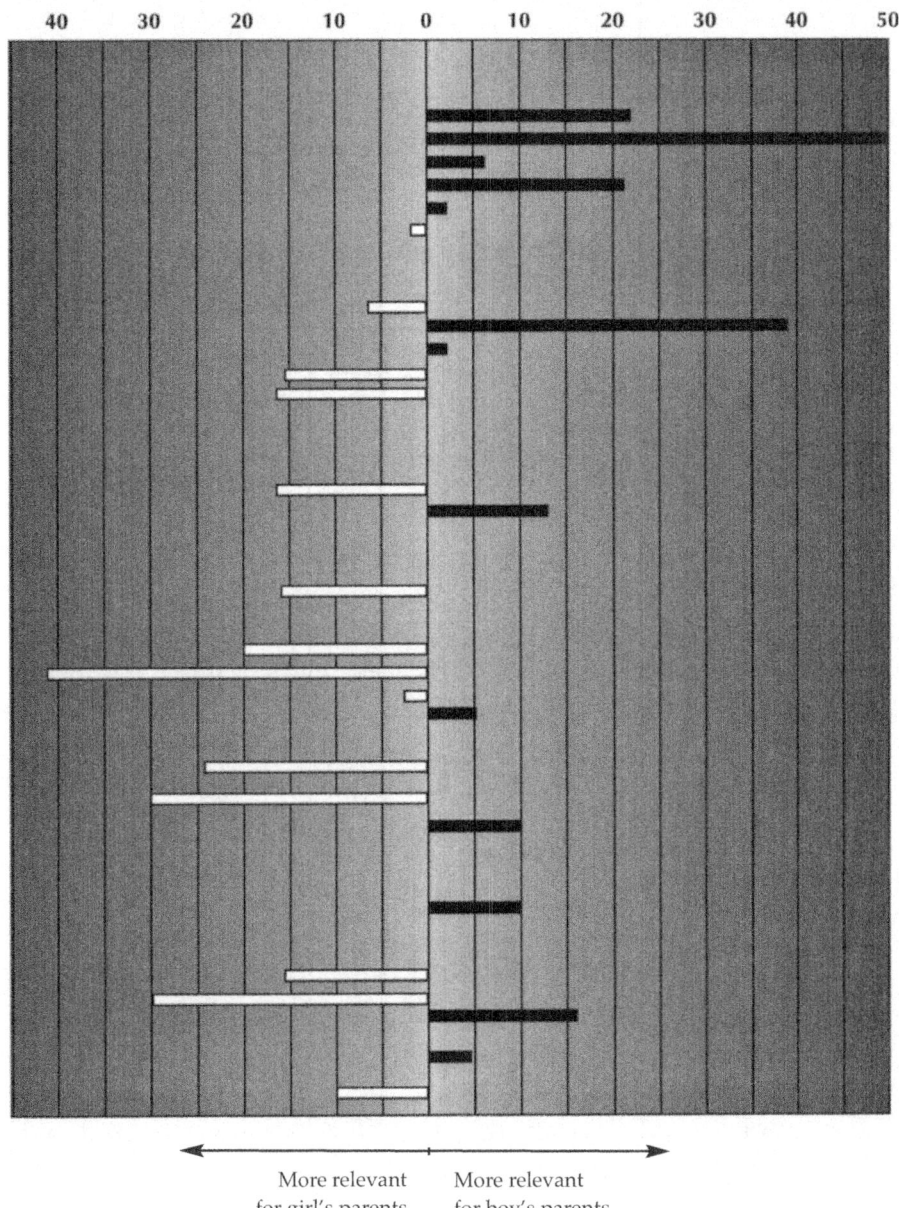

More relevant for girl's parents   More relevant for boy's parents

ACKNOWLEDGMENT

The authors gratefully acknowledge the help of Julie Busch, B.Sc., in the analysis of the data. This paper was prepared with the assistance of Medical Publications, The Hospital for Sick Children.

REFERENCES

BLOCK, R., AND RASH, F. (1981). *Handbook of behavioral pediatrics*. Chicago: Yearbook Medical Publishers, pp. 57, 77.

CORBIN, C., AND NIX, C. (1979). Sex-typing of physical activities and success predictions of children before and after cross-sex competition. *Journal of Sport Psychology* 1: 43-52.

Croce, R., and Lavay, B. (1987). Now more than ever: Physical education for the elementary school-aged child. *Runner* 25 (4) Winter: 7-1L

GRACE, N. (1987). Sports medicine section position paper: School physical education program. *Ontario Medical Review* 54 (3) March: 218-221.

HANSEN, H., AND MCKENZIE, L. (1988). Needs, benefits, barriers, change strategies, politics. Quality, daily physical education-is it possible? *CAHPER Journal* 54 (2) Mar/Apr: 29-38.

KIRKENDALL, D. (1986). Effects of physical activity on intellectual development and academic performance. In G. Stull, and H. Eckert (eds). *Effects of physical activity on children. The American Academy of Physical Education Papers, No. 19, 57th Annual Meeting, Atlanta, Georgia, April 15-16, 1985*. Champaign, IL: Human Kinetics Publishers, pp. 49-63.

KONZAK, B., AND BOUDREAU, F. (1984). Martial arts training and mental health: An exercise in self-help. *Canada's Mental Health* 32 (4) December: 2-7.

LEVINE, M., AND SATZ, P. (1984). *Middle childhood: Development and dysfunction*. Baltimore: University Park Press.

LEVINE, M., CAREY, W., CROCKER, A., ET AL. (1983). *Developmental-behavioral pediatrics*. Philadelphia: W. B. Saunders.

MILLER, R. (1989). Effects of sports instruction on children's self-concept. *Percept Motor Skills* 68: 239-242.

NOSANCHUK, T., AND MACNEIL, M. (1989). Examination of the effects of traditional and modern martial arts training on aggressiveness. *Aggressive Behaviour*, 15: 153-159.

SHAW, L., LEVINE, M., AND BELFER, M. (1982). Developmental double jeopardy: A study of clumsiness and self esteem in children with learning problems. *JDBP* 3: 191-196.

SHEPHARD, R. (1982). *Physical activity and growth*. Chicago: Year Book Medical Publishers.

SINCLAIR, G. (1983). A daily physical education pilot project. *CAHPER* 49 (Supplement) March: 22-26.

TAYLOR, J. (1986). Surviving the challenge. *Journal of Physical Education, Recreation, and Dance*, 57: 69-72.

chapter 2

Viewing Human Conflict Through the Martial Arts: Interview with Dr. Terrance Webster-Doyle

by Elisa Hendrey, M.A.

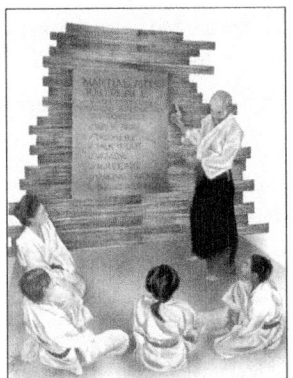 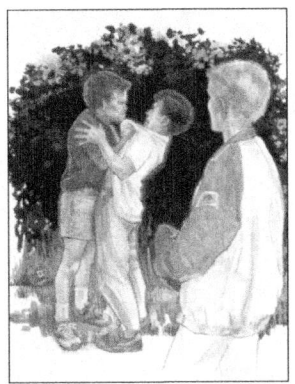

All photographs courtesy of T. Webster-Doyle.
Illustrations by Rod Cameron.

Introduction

Responsible martial arts instructors attempt in some way to teach students that their skills are to be used only for self-defense. However, Dr. Terrence Webster-Doyle, sixth dan in Take Nami-do karate, is unique in his use of the martial arts as a focus for the exploration of the actual nature of conflict itself. From his study of conflict, Webster-Doyle has developed and published an extensive Martial Arts for Peace curriculum designed to stimulate the instructor's and student's inquiries into the nature of conflict and the possibilities for peaceful conflict resolution through role-playing, games, and a variety of other structured activities that can be integrated into martial arts classes for young people. Integration of the physical skills of the martial artist combined with an understanding of conflict create what Webster-Doyle terms integrative martial arts.

Webster-Doyle believes that the purpose of the martial arts, historically, when they incorporated the "*Do*" or "the Way," was to help students do what he is attempting in the martial arts school today, that is, explore the roots of conflict that lie in conditioned thinking and action. It is his view that this was the intent of the martial arts, especially karate, with its emphasis on "empty self." Webster-Doyle's integrated, holistic approach views martial arts instruction as an educational endeavor that goes beyond just a sport or physical self-defense in an effort to shed light on the causes of conflict in all of its forms throughout the world and to find a solution to modern day violence. Giving visual testimony to Webster-Doyle's more than thirty-five years of dedication to the cause of peace is a photo taped to the wall of his Middlebury, Vermont, office. The photograph shows a young Bosnian boy inside a bus, his hands pressed against the window, tears rolling down his face as he looks out at a pair of hands, most likely his mother's, pressing toward him from the other side of the glass. The photo caption reads, "Reaching Out to the Children of Bosnia." Webster-Doyle has written "world" in place of Bosnia and beneath the photo has penned in and circled the words, "promises to keep." He explained his use of the phrase from the popular Robert Frost poem, "Stopping By Woods on a Snowy Evening," that ends with the lines, "I have promises to keep/And miles to go before I sleep." For Webster-Doyle, the poem serves as a reminder that he has made a promise to the children of the world to do all that he can to help people understand how to resolve conflict peacefully.

The following interview was conducted in Middlebury, Vermont, in October 1996.

INTERVIEW

• WHAT ARE YOU ATTEMPTING TO DO WITH THE WORK THAT YOU TERM "MARTIAL ARTS FOR PEACE"?

I'm emphasizing the whole of karate, not just doing the physical karate alone.

• COULD YOU ELABORATE A BIT ON WHAT YOU MEAN BY "THE WHOLE OF KARATE?"

Yes. An educated human being like Funakoshi Gichin, for example, who founded Shotokan Karate, looked at the art as a whole. He, for example, studied it as a complete way of life. Ninety-eight percent of what is done in the martial arts today is physical, and perhaps only two percent is understanding the philosophical concepts that are behind the art. The history of tying a sash (*obi*) has little practical application to the tremendous problem of violence in the world. What is needed is to really study conflict as one studies with tremendous effort the things that you really want to know, such as curing cancer or ending hunger. I'm taking seriously the charge I have as a martial artist, as I've been doing for the past thirty-five years.

- WHAT DO YOU MEAN WHEN YOU WAY THAT YOU ARE TAKING YOUR CHARGE AS A MARTIAL ARTIST SERIOUSLY?

The charge of the martial artist is to understand conflict—individual and global—which is created by the destructive conditioning of the brain. That's the essence—*kara-te* as empty-self. That's the crux, to be free of, empty of, this negative conditioning in the human brain. This understanding is already there historically in the martial arts literature, and I'm making it more available in a modern way. I'm examining the structure of psychological conditioning that creates the isolated ego or fragmented self and putting it in a context that our young people can understand so they can begin to comprehend what effects this conditioning has in creating not only on the playground but also in what we call war. As it existed, it was hard for them to understand; it was intellectual and esoteric.

- WHAT DO YOU BELIEVE WAS THE INTENTION OF THE EARLY MARTIAL ARTISTS IN REGARD TO VIOLENCE AND RESOLVING CONFLICT?

The founders of the martial arts were important figures pointing the way to understanding the nature and structure of human conflict, but now we have to look into the matter of conflict scientifically, objectively. It's a real study. I should say, though, that not all of the founders agreed. I think Funakoshi, as an educator, looked at the martial arts more as a whole endeavor toward a way of life that encompassed the relationship of human beings to each other, a way of life that was intelligent, that allowed people to bring an intelligent approach to dealing with conflict. Remember, Funakoshi studied, wrote poetry, appreciated the arts. He didn't consider karate a sport at all.

- WHAT, SPECIFICALLY, DO YOU ATTEMPT TO TEACH CHILDREN SO THAT THEY CAN USE THEIR MARTIAL ART TO RESOLVE CONFLICT WITHOUT VIOLENCE?

I teach them to A.R.M. themselves. That is, to Avoid conflict by preventing it; to Resolve conflict through what I call "mental self-defense," that is, nonviolent alternatives; and to Manage conflict by the humane application of physical skills if need be. But one hopes that the first two "lines of defense," so to speak, will allow the individual to stop conflict before it becomes physical.

- ARE THERE EXERCISES, GAMES OR ACTIVITIES THAT YOU USE TO TEACH THESE CONCEPTS TO CHILDREN?

Yes, there are martial arts "games" I do, for instance, when I teach conflict avoidance or prevention. First, I talk to the students about the energy that is around them that they can't see, taste or touch. Then I walk toward them until they tell me to stop because they are uncomfortable. I ask them how it feels when I violate their space.

In the second activity, I put someone in the center of a circle with his or her eyes closed. Another student who is part of the circle walks toward the one in the center. With a heightened sensitivity to a threat, the student in the center, who cannot see, responds to the approach by pointing to the invader. Then we discuss the activity so that the students can understand the importance of being aware.

In the third game, called "Friend or Foe," we are reading body language. Some police departments use a form of this game with a big screen and a laser gun. When we play the game, one individual walks up to a student with the intention of either shaking hands or punching. The student must attempt to tell from body language what the intent is, because he or she must either block or shake hands. This activity teaches students to respond correctly to either a friendly or threatening situation.

- SO YOU BEGIN WITH PREVENTION AND BUILD THE STUDENT'S ABILITY TO INCREASE AND DEVELOP AWARENESS?

Yes. It involves a layering of skills. The next part is to learn to resolve conflict mentally. This is the secondary level in which we do bully/victim roles. I help students develop soliloquies that are like mental katas. For any threatening situation they should have at least three alternatives in case one doesn't work. The parallel in the martial arts is to be able to do multiple blocks and moves in order to avoid injury. The instructor is there to ask the students what would work and what wouldn't work. I give suggestions. The instructor has to be flexible in this role.

- AND WHAT DOES THE THIRD LEVEL, MANAGING CONFLICT, INVOLVE?

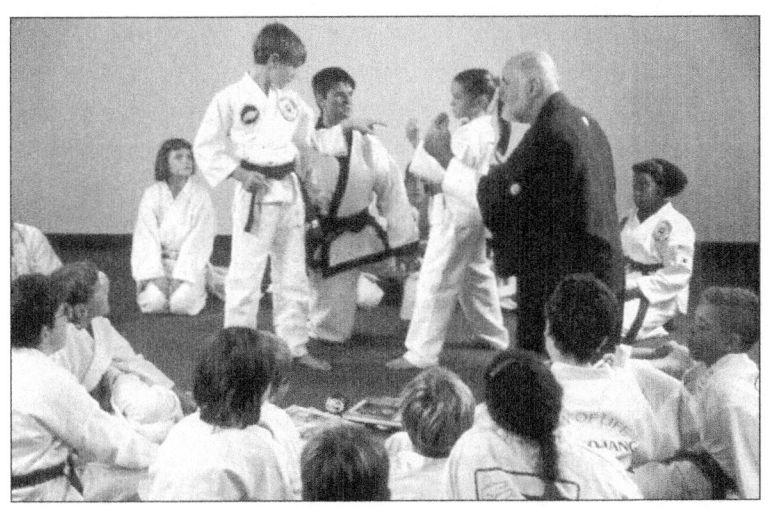

There are self-defense skills one would need for protection, but there is more than just those skills. The physical level of managing conflict is not just self-defense. Students have to integrate the physical and mental at this point, too. Remember, one of the terms I use to describe what I'm attempting to teach is "integrative martial arts." A narrow focus, for instance, on repetitions of too many self-defense patterns makes the body rigid. This is why I use Shu-ha-ri.

Shu-ha-ri is a traditional martial arts concept. It literally means: *Shu*—learning from tradition; *Ha*—insight; *Ri*—transcendence or going beyond. It signifies the learning process. In the physical art it means learning basic, traditional forms, which is Shu. I teach basic forms to give the student a foundation. Then I develop with each student his or her own unique form or kata. This is Ha, which gives the students insight into themselves. Then we do the Ri forms, which are the most difficult yet the most exciting. This is when a student does a spontaneous free form. He or she stands, bows and then performs a form, a kata that is totally improvisational, free, unlike the prescribed forms of Shu. The kata can last a brief minute or last for a good length of time. It is up to each student. This form is only done once, then it is gone.

Learning all levels of Shu-ha-ri gives the student not only the traditional foundation, which is necessary, but also a personalized form tailored for him or her, and then the freedom of spontaneous, unprescribed movement. In this way, we are not a victim of rote conditioning, physically or mentally. We have the breaking up of the traditional with Ha and Ri but at the same time we don't "throw the baby out with the bath water," as the saying goes.

- EVEN IF YOU DO NOT WANT TO OVER-EMPHASIZE REPETITION OF PATTERNS, I KNOW THAT YOU BELIEVE THAT ATTAINING THE PHYSICAL SKILLS OF A MARTIAL ART IS OF GREAT VALUE IN HELPING THE INDIVIDUAL TO REACT TO CONFLICT IN A MANNER THAT ALLOWS ALTERNATIVES TO THE FIGHT-OR-FLIGHT REACTION. WOULD YOU EXPLAIN HOW THIS WORKS?

You see, we seem to have an either/or society. Either fight or run. The conventional approaches to resolving conflict don't work because of this fight-or-flight reaction, which is a conditioned response, which may be appropriate in certain situations, but it is generally an inappropriate reaction. The body is conditioned to react unnecessarily to a situation. This type of conditioning pervades the whole education of the child—to react habitually, mentally or physically, to a situation.

Where the martial arts come in is that if I know I have the ability to fight, then I don't have to use flight. If I'm untrained, the message to my brain is, "I gotta get out of here." But to the martial artist, the message is that, "this is a threat, but I can deal with it." Then you can be taught verbal, nonviolent alternatives like the "Twelve Ways To Walk Away With Confidence" that I use in my curriculum and in my books to get out of the situation. My father was a firefighter, and my father wasn't afraid to go in to fight fire because he was trained. It's the same thing with the martial arts and conflict.

- YOU USE "THE TWELVE WAY TO WALK AWAY WITH CONFIDENCE" IN YOUR CLASSES. WHAT ARE SOME OTHER MENTAL ACTIVITIES YOU USE?

To show young people how individual conflict escalates into global conflict, I take a two-sided map into the martial arts class. On one side is the physical representation of the Earth. There's no writing on it. The children know what it is. I ask them what they see, and they see just what is there. The other side, the political side, is broken up into countries, tribal territories. From outer space the Earth is not broken up when you look at it. The mind breaks it up. That's the ethnocentric tribal mode of thinking. The children understand this. To them it is simple, uncomplicated. Yet they, at their age, don't understand all the implications of this.

Everything I do in a martial arts class is to demonstrate the conditioned mind, and I always tell the children to question what I say. Everything in the dojo or school can be used to create tools for educating about conditioning. I make a child a black belt for the day. Then I ask, "How did you feel with a black belt?" The students say, "awesome," "powerful." Then I hold the belt up. What do you see? The children say, "power," "strength." Then someone says, "It's just cloth." That's a lesson about conditioned thinking, that there is just what something is and there is what we believe it to be.

Students often say that a martial art is just physical self-defense and an art form. But it should also be a vehicle for self-understanding. I ask, for example, if students are aware of tension in their bodies. They have a rigid posture. They're uptight, but they'll ask me what I mean. They may take it as a judgment. That's a defense mechanism. However, if I ask, "What is your body telling you," they'll be able to tell me because I am asking what they are feeling, which is not taken as a judgment of them or of their behavior. It is the judgment that creates the defenses and the conditioning.

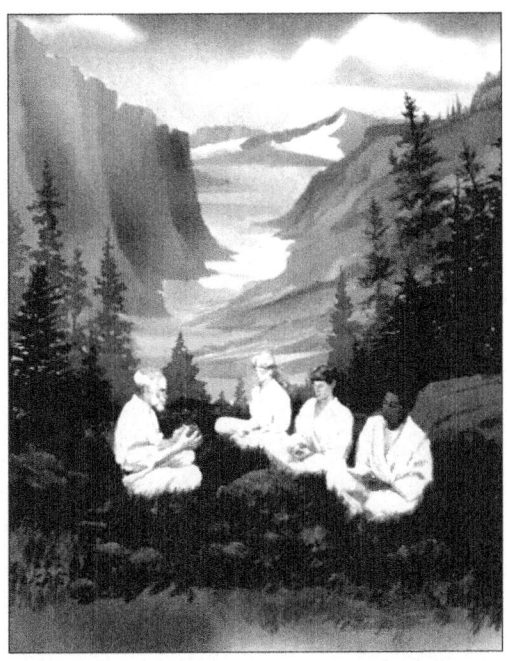

- WOULD YOU REJECT ALL CONDITIONED RESPONSES?

The concept of Shu-ha-ri is very important here. You need a questioning mind, but this doesn't mean that you reject something on its face value.

Some conditioning is necessary. We are conditioned to put the foot on the brake to stop the car. That's a correct reaction. We are conditioned to block and punch. That's good, to a point. If we use only traditional forms, however, we can be out guessed by our opponents and lose in free-style because they have figured out our methods. On the other hand, thousands of years of ethnocentric tribal conditioning have been handed down to us and with it the physical/psychological reactions that worked then for survival. That was good then, but now it's working against us. The psychological identity with the group or tribe is creating physical conflict today. At one time, identifying with a group or tribe was necessary for insuring physical survival, so the individual identity became the group or tribal identity and vice-versa. At this point, psychological identification became the means to insure physical survival. The "me," or "self" or ego became the identity associated with the group. "I" am "us." And "us" is "me." This identification as the isolated ethnocentric identity "me/we" now creates conflict and prevents physical security, whereas at one time it insured it. Bosnia is an example.

- OBVIOUSLY, YOU BELIEVE THAT PEOPLE CAN BE TAUGHT TO OVERCOME CONDITIONED REACTIONS THAT CREATE CONFLICT OR PREVENT THE PEACEFUL RESOLUTION OF CONFLICT.

Yes. In martial arts, we're trying to open the child's mind to looking into this form of conditioning. Children learn to hate and fear. Watch children being raised to hate each other in Northern Ireland, the Middle East or wherever. If I am told something over and over for a period of time and I believed or acted without questioning, then I was conditioned. Tell a Serb over a period of time that a Muslim is an enemy, and he believes it. This is where martial art becomes very important. Let's look at how the brain reacts to a potentially hostile situation.

In the case of ethnocentric identification, a person from one faction sees the other as a potential enemy. At the root of the problem, the brain is reacting to a basic instinctual threat to its physical well being even though the threat is only psychological.

Now how do the martial arts help? If there is a threat or a supposed threat, it goes into the brain, and if the child doesn't have the physical skills to fight or run away with confidence, he will react in a fight/flight manner. With physical skills, however, the message goes into the brain, and the child thinks, "Oh, I can deal with this." The fight-or-flight instinct just needs assurance that it can fight, it has the martial art training, if it needs to fight. Then the child can deal more rationally with the situation than without the physical martial art skill. It's like tricking the brain, the fight/flight reaction. Then there is an opportunity for an intelligent response instead of an inappropriate reaction. Now with this biologically conditioned reaction in a state of abeyance, one can act from understanding, from intelligence.

- Do you believe there are martial arts instructors and parents of martial arts students who would resist your focus on nonviolent resolution of conflict?

Well, peace is frightening because it means letting down defenses. It reminds me of the novel, *1984*. There is a deep negative conditioning at work in that novel. One has to think in stereotypical ways in the society described in the novel. There's a seeming safety in that kind of thinking—a tribal notion. But, in fact, this reverting to tribalism just compounds the problem and creates more conflict.

- Understanding conflict and the role of conditioning sounds rather complex. How difficult is it to teach children about these concepts?

The greatest myth is that only the authority on a subject can understand it. The average person can understand the concepts I'm dealing with. We created conflict, so we can understand it. It's not so difficult as we've made it. I know that a young person ten to fourteen years of age can understand the basic concept of conflict. And it's not that difficult to understand conditioning. It's quite straight forward, as I explained with the example of tribalism. If we begin to understand the foundation, the nature and structure of conflict, of conditioned thinking and action, we can end it there. It is when it gets to the level of politics and the like that it gets complicated.

- Is there any place where your ideas are being taught to children?

Yes. Dr. Mike Foley, an expert martial artist, someone who understands what I'm doing, has used the "Bully Program" at private and public schools in Phoenix, Arizona. And my ideas are being used at our Martial Arts for Peace School in the same area, which is being operated temporarily out of a local center by a family of martial artists, the Contreras family.

- What is the "Bully Program"?

It involves role-playing. It defines what a bully is, what a victim is, how they portray those characteristics in their body language, how to understand and avoid being a bully or a victim at what I call the primary level that I spoke of earlier when I explained A.R.M. The primary or avoidance level is prevention.

The program uses "The Twelve Ways To Walk Away With Confidence," and it employs lots of games, stories, and role-plays for young people. The program has also been used in elementary grades and in junior high schools in the public school system throughout the U.S. and internationally. Many martial arts schools use this program successfully, too.

I should add that the "Bully Program" talks about many different types of bullies, such as the whiner bully as well as the aggressive bullies. Also, the bullies who are accepted by society—the patriotic bullies and the business bullies, for example. The same basic structure underlies all bullies, however. The program also teaches relationship skills, not only how to protect oneself from bullies but how to get what one wants without becoming a bully. These are social skills.

• WHAT WAS THE OUTCOME OF THE "BULLY PROGRAM" WHERE IT WAS USED IN ARIZONA? YOU DID A STUDY IN ONE OF THE PRIVATE SCHOOLS THERE, DID YOU NOT?

The result was that kids became more assertive and less aggressive, but I want to do the program in a martial arts school and do a study there. I've seen kids change, even radically change, in just a summer. The physical aspect of the martial art gets the young people in the door. Then the mental aspect changes them. Some of these kids had been on the edge of getting into real trouble. Now they do beautiful katas. They have good manners now.

• WHAT HAPPENS WHEN ONLY THE PHYSICAL ASPECT OF THE MARTIAL ARTS IS TAUGHT?

It actually compounds the problem of violence. Teaching the physical only reinforces the code that "might is right." Recently I did a workshop at a large martial arts school in Massachusetts, and one of the children said, "Show me your martial arts," meaning, show me the physical. I said, "I've been doing it all the time," which meant that I had been showing the students the mental martial arts.

In teaching only the physical, you are teaching no other line of defense. In my teaching, for instance with the "Twelve Ways To Walk Away With Confidence," the first line of defense is avoid. I am lessening the odds of a physical confrontation. But there are no guarantees. I am increasing the alternatives, however. If students are taught only the physical, the children will only know that. Then there are no other options.

• I HAVE HEARD YOU USE THE TERM "HOLISTIC APPROACH" IN REGARD TO YOUR

CONCEPTS. WHAT DO YOU MEAN WHEN YOU SAY THIS?

Martial Arts for Peace, as I call it, does work in the sense of lessening the odds of violent conflict because it is holistic. It includes the three levels of dealing with conflict that I term the primary, secondary and tertiary. Tertiary (physical) skills help you not to go into a fight-or-flight state, so there is a state of abeyance, and then the individual can think. This thinking comes from the primary and secondary levels, how to avoid or resolve conflict nonviolently. As a whole, the techniques I use work, but they have to be taught. The instruction has to be balanced. We have to spend much more time, not just ten minutes of a class, teaching these skills. This is so very important to understand!

- IS IT PRACTICAL TO SPEND A LARGER PORTION OF TIME THAN TEN MINUTES PER CLASS ON NONPHYSICAL TECHNIQUES AND STRATEGIES?

It's not only practical but necessary. Children have to be able to cope with conflict. It has to be a priority, because we see the importance of it for ourselves. I don't want to just talk about conflict. I care about really understanding it and dealing with it. International conflict and conflict on the playground have the same structure. We must see that participating in the martial art is a potential way to understand human conflict.

With young people I do a lesson using a model plastic human head. We pretend we are developing a human being and we are going to put things into the head. The human needs to know how to get home—practical knowledge. We put that information in the head. What about hurt feelings? Pain and anger? The children say "No, don't put those in." They don't want them. Do you have those things in your brain, I ask them. "Yes," they say. "How did they get there," I ask. Someone tells me that they get there by someone putting them there. The fears that are there, everything that's there was put there. That's conditioning, inappropriate unquestioned information. With this example we show them the difference between necessary and useful knowledge and knowledge that creates conflict.

So, how do we get the negative conditioning out that we don't want? Thinking is the creator of the problem. Can thinking solve the problem that it created? I use awareness exercises to enhance observation. I walk toward them. I ask them to tell me to stop when they are uncomfortable. This is awareness. Then we turn it inward after a while to be aware of our brain, to observe our thinking, in action. It's simple but profound.

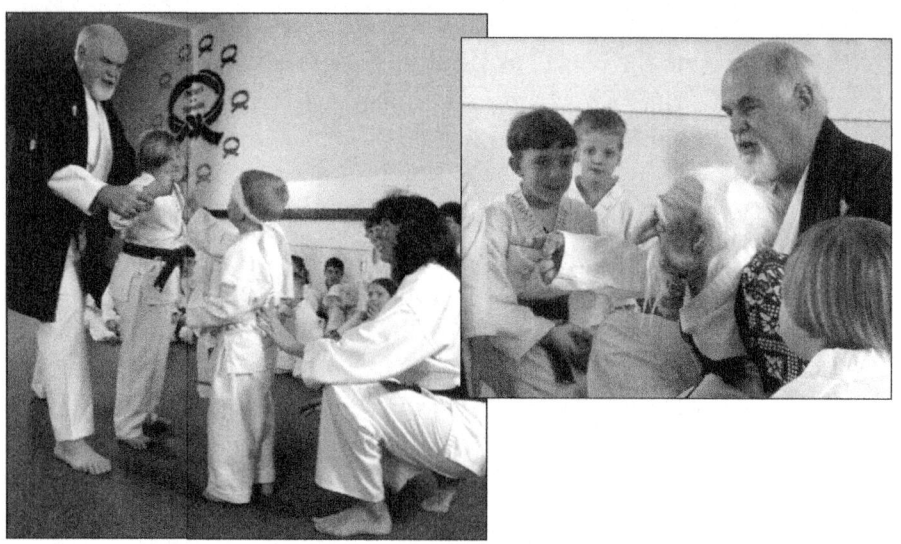

Another exercise involves blindfolding one child. One child leads another child around. The child who is being led touches things. He jumps when his hands are put in lukewarm water, which is the last thing in the exercise that the child touches. But when the blindfold is taken off and the exercise is repeated without it, the child doesn't jump when his hands are put in water. His jumping the first time showed a feeling like, "Oh, wow!" It's a newness of feeling, like going to the ocean for the first time—a pleasant surprise. But when they know that it is "just" water, the excitement is gone. This is where boredom comes from. We don't see a day as new.

The conditioning that I want them to see is the same basic structure involved in any conditioning. It's the same structure that leads to war. That's a quantum leap, but children can understand conditioning at this simpler level first.

They have a prejudgment—conditioning. This shows in the extreme what creates war; this shows what prejudice is, prejudgment of saying, I know what you are, you're a such and such. We must enhance children's awareness and insight. That's learning. Accumulated learning is one kind. Learning what's happening at the moment, through observation, is another kind.

- THERE IS CLEARLY A GREAT DEAL TO TEACH IN THE AREAS OF THE MENTAL PART OF MARTIAL ARTS TRAINING AS YOU ENVISION IT. HOW WOULD YOU IDEALLY ALLOT CLASS TIME?

One half hour physical, and one half hour mental.

- YOU HAVE WRITTEN A SERIES OF BOOKS FOR CHILDREN WHO STUDY MARTIAL ARTS THAT ARE DESIGNED TO BE USED IN MARTIAL ARTS SCHOOLS. DO YOU HAVE A PERSONAL FAVORITE AMONG THEM?

Tug of War and *Fighting the Invisible Enemy* are my best and most important ones. The latter deals with the essence of the martial arts, that being its potential for stopping conflict. It asks, "What is conflict," and it looks at the essential part that conditioning plays in conflict. That book really introduces children to what conditioning and conflict are. The child—any human being—needs to know the role that conditioning plays in conflict.

When I was younger and heard the words "women's liberation," I had a physical reaction. I was conditioned. I'm not trying to say what a right relationship is or what is peace, but I just want to understand what creates conflict and therefore what prevents peace. This is a very important distinction.

Wanting peace leads to ideals and, therefore, one is conditioned to act in peaceful ways according to some philosophy. And others are conditioned to act peacefully according to other viewpoints, depending on their background. This is all based on judgment of the fact that one is violent. The logical reaction is to be peaceful. But "peaceful" according to whose or which viewpoint? The conditioning starts with the judgment of conflict being "bad" and peace being "good," which is the structure and nature of conditioned thinking. This is looking at the fundamental root of the problem of conflict. We are trying to "solve" it through intellectual means alone without observing the actual fact of conflict. This book introduces questioning in place of assuming that one is behaving correctly.

Tug of War deals with the extreme outcome of conflict: war. For one thing, it deals with double-speak, the way we use language so that it desensitizes us to conflict. A very important chapter deals with how we create an enemy in our own minds. I think it's factual, not just my opinion. Those two books working together are very powerful.

Another part of *Tug of War* deals with why we react as we do. This is the book that talks about how thousands of years ago people needed to come together in groups to survive and how this created psychological identity that has been passed on down through time, starting from a tribal belief and ritual and resulting in custom and tradition. We've become conditioned, so now the psychological image triggers the biological flight-or-fight reaction. One is preparing to fight a supposed threat.

These books work even for children as young as six through eight years of age. The books are like flowers developing from buds. They can be read over and over through the years, and there will be an unfolding like a flower for the reader.

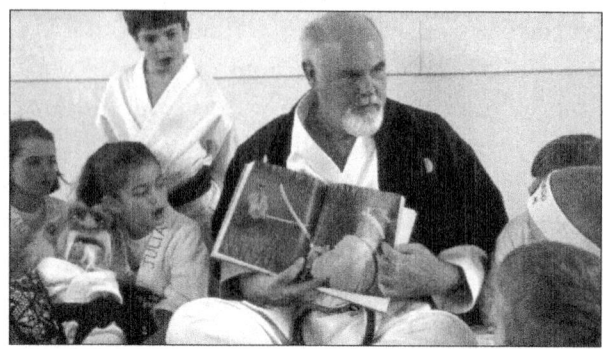

- IN SOME OF YOUR BOOKS, YOU USE FAMILIAR ASIAN STORIES. WHY HAVE YOU TURNED TO THESE OLD TALES?

The old Asian stories are in the books because they're really good. I took them and made them modern for young people and adults in *The Eye of the Hurricane* and the other Martial Arts for Peace books. These stories have good insights into human nature, and we must preserve them, but students must see the practical in them. That's what Europeans and Americans haven't done. Those stories were all reflections of a state of mind—the real basics—and they have to come back. Then the physical art will have a proper context within which to be practiced.

- YOU'VE ALSO BEGUN WRITING A COLUMN FOR CHILDREN ON A REGULAR BASIS IN *KARATE/KUNG FU ILLUSTRATED*. WHAT ARE YOUR GOALS FOR THE COLUMN?

I've been writing in "Black Belt for Kids" for more than a year now. The column appears every other month as an insert in the magazine. Many of the stories question whether knowledge alone can solve problems of conflict or whether it compounds it. I use an example from my children's book *Breaking the Chains of the Ancient Warrior*. I ask the children to tell me what they think order is, knowing that whatever they say will not be order. I say to them that whatever their answer is, it cannot be true. This is a real story. They all gave me explanations except for a seven-year-old boy, Oliver, who pointed to all of my books lined up on the shelves but said nothing. I said, "That's right." He had given an example of order. When I asked them again to tell me what they knew about order, they then ran around the room and straightened it up. But when I suddenly called, "Line up," they all pushed and shoved to get in line. They said that they had forgotten about order when I confronted them at this point as to why they had reverted back to disorder. So, I asked them if only knowing about order brings about order, and they said, "No, Sensei." They lined up again. "Be aware," I told them. "Look right, look left. Do it, don't tell me!"

Most intellectuals think that learning about peace creates it, but it creates conflicts. We each get our own idea of it, and then we're in conflict. Knowledge about peace compounds the problems, but insight doesn't. So, certain forms of knowledge are destructive.

- TO WHOM DO YOU THINK YOUR IDEAS HAVE THE MOST APPEAL?

I don't appeal to the intellectuals because they want to make this a Tibetan Buddhist meditation practice or something like that, and I don't appeal to some others because they don't want to look at themselves; they think that the martial arts are only physical. So I appeal to children.

I'm not inventing something new. When Funakoshi said, "empty-self," he was really saying something. It is this "empty-self," *kara-te*, that is the foundation of all martial arts. It is a universal insight, revealing the roots of conflict. Karate is not just a physical self-defense.

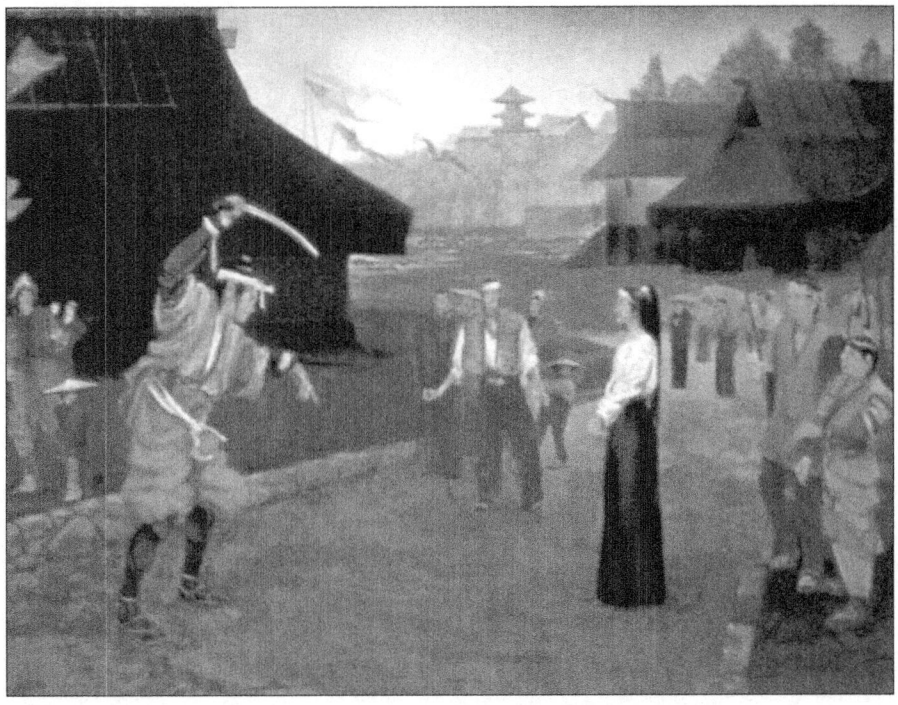

- **What do you see as necessary skills in a Martial Arts for Peace instructor?**

Teachers must have patience and a good sense of humor. I feel like we're pioneers. With so many children studying martial arts, we need to have comprehensive understanding of conflict as well as excellent physical skills. Some instructors with good intentions talk to students about not fighting, but there is not much depth to it. We can stop this human butchering. It is resolvable, but to do it, we must understand what is in us, and not create an ideal of peace.

- **I know that your martial arts background includes your Gensei-Ryu training up to a nidan under Shigeru Numano, who came to America in 1966, and that you've studied several other styles as well, dating back to the 1950's. I understand that you also founded a style that you named Take Nami-Do, the Way of the Bamboo and Wave. Why did you decide to start your own style?**

I founded it, not that I wanted to found a style, but it came about because in Gensei-ryu there wasn't an emphasis on the mental. I asked myself, "dare I," and I did. But then I dropped it. I thought I wanted to have an intention, not teach another style. So my patch says Martial Arts for Peace.

I just want to be a teacher of the martial arts, the art of kara-te, of empty-self. By karate, I don't just mean the physical art but rather the practical philosophy of "empty-self," of understanding what prevents peace, what creates conflict.

- **What is your background in the field of education, outside of the martial arts?**

I have a Masters in psychology and a Ph.D. in health and human resources and have taught philosophy, education, and psychology at the university level, and I've worked in juvenile delinquency prevention. My wife Jean and I founded the Atrium School in California, where the focus of the high school curriculum was on understanding and resolving conflict. Someday we both want to start a martial arts high school, just like a traditional school but with martial arts as a basis for self-understanding.

- **And the curriculum guides that you've developed include one specifically for use in martial arts schools, and the other for use in public and private schools?**

Yes, that's right.

- CAN YOU BRIEFLY DESCRIBE YOUR ROLE IN THE MARTIAL ARTS FOR PEACE ASSOCIATION AND THE SHUHARI INSTITUTE?

I'm the founder and director of the Martial Arts for Peace Association, which is headquartered in Middlebury, Vermont, and I established the Shuhari Institute, which is dedicated to achieving peace by understanding conflict through the study of the martial arts. It is the research and development branch of the association.

- WHAT IS YOUR VISION OF MARTIAL ARTS EDUCATION IN THE FUTURE?

I'd like to see the martial arts for the twenty-first century be martial arts as education. There's the martial arts self-defense instructor, the coach for tournaments, and that's fine. I have nothing against tournaments, but there is also the martial arts educator. What I'd like to see develop is how martial arts can teach healthy values, healthy social behavior. I'd like to see four years of a martial arts high school and then a martial arts college with an instructors' college, too.

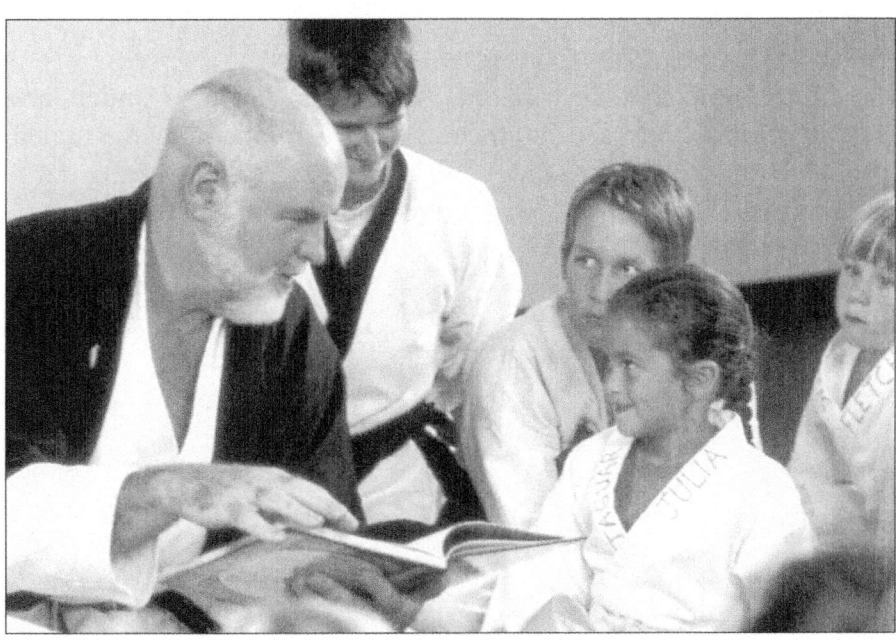

- YOU MENTIONED A MARTIAL ARTS CODE OF CONDUCT. YOU ALREADY HAVE PUBLISHED A CURRICULUM FOR MARTIAL ARTS SCHOOLS TO USE IN TEACHING THIS CODE, I BELIEVE.

Yes, it has a wide variety of activities to use with children and includes topics like the manner of the week, respect and the like. It is not a "code" in the strict sense of the word but rather like Shu of Shu-ha-ri, a foundation by which young people can explore traditional values in an intelligent, questioning manner. Through this inquiry, young people can come to an understanding of ethics, of values, through their own exploration. Then values will not be imposed upon them, conditioned into them, without question. Of course, it depends on the age of the child. I'm not advocating license to do anything they want. Neither am I advocating a strict, unbending "code" that they are supposed to follow obediently just because we adults say they should. It's really just a mixture of good common sense and democratic thinking.

- MOST OF WHAT WE'VE DISCUSSED TODAY HAS FOCUSED ON CHILDREN. DO YOU WORK WITH ADULTS?

Yes, I provide workshops for children and adults, but I'm particularly committed to working with young people and those who deal with young people to help them understand conflict and find ways to resolve conflict peacefully.

- WHAT WOULD YOU SAY IS YOUR ULTIMATE GOAL?

I'm bound and determined as a human being to understand human conflict, and I see that the martial arts have a potential to help people understand and resolve conflict peacefully. I'm reaching out to the children of the world. I have promises to keep.

chapter 3

Kon and Haku:
The Spirit of Heaven and Earth in Children[1]

by Sakuyama Yoshinaga, B.A., translated by Duncan Robert Mark[2]

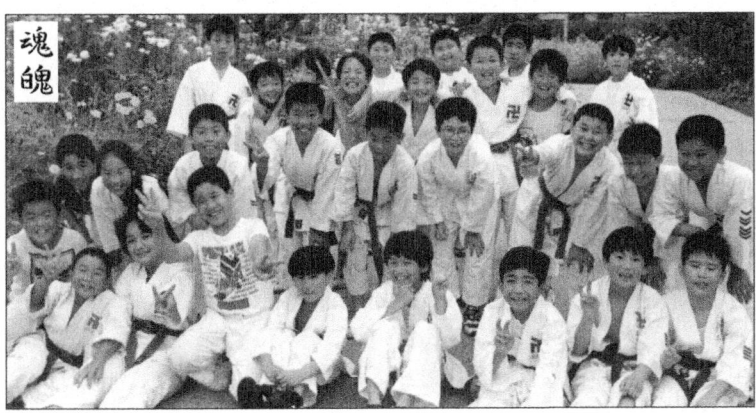

Desire

    I once took part in an organized fast. We went for four days without food. On the fifth day, we got thinned noodle soup. The old woman who sat next to me said that it was delicious, and cried. It really was so delicious as to bring one to tears. This experience led me to understand that the more you desire something, the more you value what you get. Education is the same. It is impossible to appreciate learning when knowledge is being forced into objecting students. If you desire to learn, then you will find ways to learn. It is the teachers who have to inspire students to desire to learn.

---

[1] *Kon* is the part of the spirit which is separate from the flesh and is thought to return to heaven when one dies. *Haku* is the part of the spirit which resides in the flesh and is thought to return to the earth when one dies.

[2] First published in Japanese under the title "Developing Kon and Haku" in *Gekkan Budo* (1998, September).

The other day I went to a high school reunion. I hadn't seen most of my classmates for over thirty years and everyone had gotten quite a bit older. For quite some time, I didn't recognize Mr. Izawa, who used to be in charge, sitting next to me. I apologized to him for my impoliteness at the same time being glad to see him. I was glad to have the chance to thank him after thirty years.

I have been fortunate enough to have opened an English language school and have had many opportunities to travel abroad. This is entirely due to Mr. Izawa. When I was in junior high school, I was bad at and really disliked English. I was so bad at English that I was actually thrown out of an English language school. Then, when I was in the third year of high school, I suddenly had a change of heart. This was because Mr. Izawa was put in charge of the class. He told us, "Since I have been put in charge of teaching this class English, I am going to make sure you can do it a little." Having said this, he made us do fifteen minutes of composition each day before class in the time allocated for homeroom activities. This was not part of the formal teaching but something extra he devised. He said, "This is just for those who want to do it." We were to attempt to make four sentences and then take them to him. That was all. At first, I struggled. However, he never criticized me. He always gave some advice on a point and commented that I had improved.

That was a pleasure. I slowly improved. Then it became interesting. Within six months, English became my best subject. To my surprise I had come to like English.

"Make yourself devise ways of doing things." I think that this was the most exciting instruction I experienced in the whole of my school time. However, even if I mentioned this story to my classmates, none of them would remember it. It was not as significant for everybody else as it was for me. However much the teacher broadcasts, if the student does not tune into the channel, the message is not transmitted. At that time, I was probably ready to receive the teacher's broadcast. It is only when the student is ready to receive instruction that education takes place.

Growth

Based on the above experience, I will talk about the psychological development of infants. It is important to identify the stages of growth in a changing child and to nourish their psyche at the right time.

The psychological development of children takes place in roughly three stages: infancy, childhood, and adolescence. The contents at each stage differ. During the infancy and childhood periods, *kon* and *haku* are especially developed. *Kon* is the part of the spirit that is separate from the flesh and is thought to return to heaven when one dies. *Haku* is the life force, the part of the spirit that resides in the flesh and is thought to return to the earth when one dies. United, kon and haku are called *kokoro*.

1. Infancy

The life force is developed first in infancy. This life force or power to live may also be called *haku*. Children need to have experiences that develop haku. To develop haku, it is necessary to be physically active and to come into contact with other living things. This means letting children play a lot. Especially playing in the natural environment and getting feedback from it gives the opportunity to develop a feeling of oneness with nature. If you let children play in nature they will play without becoming bored. It is because the nutrition needed for life keeps flowing into them.

Walk in the woods with a child. Just that activates a child's life force. The eyes and the body start moving busily. At first they poke an insect with a dry twig, but before you know it, it is on their palm. Life energy is being exchanged. Life becomes stronger by coming into contact with life. Mountain streams and the ocean are good for this energy exchange, too. Nature is a treasury of sensual and experiential material. If haku is developed properly during this phase, one can become an adult in spite of any adverse circumstances.

2. Childhood

In the childhood stage kon, which controls haku, is developed most. Within kon, there are the emotional elements of joy, anger, sadness, pleasure, and so on, and though it is a sensitive subject the notions of good and evil are also included. If man is to live like a man then this kon must be developed. This is because kon gives directionality to haku.

Kon develops in the context of your environment. All the things that occur between friends, teachers, neighbors, and of course, family, parents, house, dogs, cats, and so on flow into kon; and for better or for worse, kon is developed. The experience of joy or peacefulness, strong love, and affection will surely develop a rich kon. Experience of challenging difficulties, perseverance, and endurance will surely develop a strong kon. However, too much pain or a strong shock may damage kon. Moreover, hateful or cowardly experiences will surely foul kon.

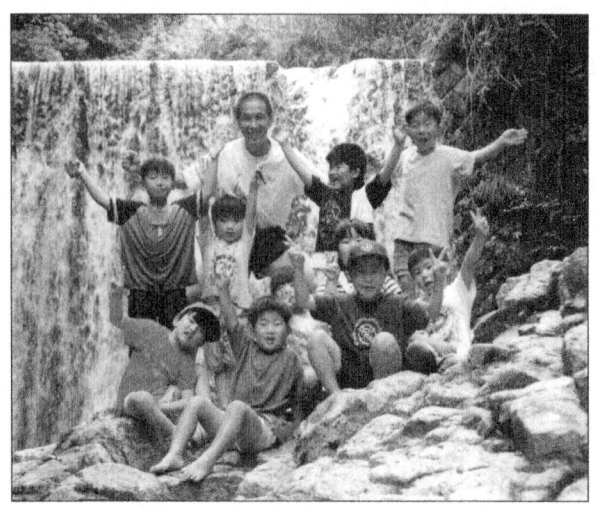

In this modern society, there is an excess of information and there are a lot of bad stimuli for children too. We adults have to provide a good environment for the development of our children's kon. Education's role in this regard is very important. With regard to the educational environment, the Japanese Education Ministry has surprisingly indicated that the "development of survival skills" is required, and the central education board has of late had "the education of the heart" at its core. The education of haku and kon has now been officially recognized.

3. Adolescence

Adolescence is when the development of the kon and haku are polished off. Also at this period, the intellectual power to understand and will power are developed the most. The awareness to act on the basis of thought is developed. Knowledge, logic, the scientific-thinking method, and so on serve as nutrition.

4. Ecdysis: "Shedding One's Skin"

The transition from infancy to childhood and from childhood to adolescence is generally known as a period of contrariness. I do not feel comfortable with this expression. I want to call it the ecdysical phase. The children are intently on their way to independence. That is what is called "growing up." To develop to the next phase, children negate the protection they have received up to that point. If the same level of protection continues, the child cannot move on to the next level in their development. For parents who wish their children to stay as they are, it may be contrariness but for the children it is a necessary ecdysis in their development. One can also experience this ecdysis in the dojo. A child that has been very obedient up to that point suddenly turns on a little joke made. In the past, I used to get angry and respond with, "What did you say?" but now I understand and I tend to think, "The time has come!"

Developing Kon and Haku

During the infancy and childhood period, the door to the heart is open. This is because the heart needs nourishment. If the heart is fed ample nourishment during this period, one will go through life with a lot of vitality and an open mind, even if one leads a largely intellectual life.

The heart is sensitively aware. It is illogical and sensual and therefore hard to express in words. Therefore, nutrition for the heart gets into it through the five senses and emotions rather than from language. One action develops the heart more than a million words.

Three years after I opened my dojo, during the children's practice, a new child threw up. All the children nearby jumped back. When I got back from the bathroom after cleaning up the child who had thrown up, the other children said things like, "Ugh. That's disgusting!" and kept their distance from the vomit. It was somewhat pitiful.

I made up my mind and began to gather together the vomit with my bare hands. There is a reason behind this. This occurred as I was cleaning an outside toilet when I was in junior high school. I was using a stick to try to poke out leaves, layers of paper, and so on that were blocking the urinal and I wasn't making much progress. One of my teachers came up and took the garbage out with his bare hands. This incident was very vivid so I remembered it. I gathered together and scooped up the vomit by hand and put it into the garbage pail. The dojo instantaneously became silent. I scooped up handfuls again and again. Then one of the children who was watching quietly said, "Teacher, I will do it, too." And he began to scoop up the vomit empty handed. Then the others joined in and scooped it up. So the whole dojo became like a cooperative workshop. Some children brought dustpans and others started cleaning with their own brand-new dusters. It was like a festival. It seemed as if a fire had been lit under the children's sleeping energy. I felt like crying. It was the first time I felt that their hearts had made a connection to each other. I realized that the heart moves other hearts through action. Moreover, I realized that once the heart is moved, it creates an enormous energy that throws reasoned judgment to the wind.

This event took place at a time when I hadn't had much experience in teaching children and I didn't have much confidence. I was able to learn a guiding principle for subsequent instruction from this small occurrence.

Teaching Shorinji Kempo

Thus my purpose in instructing children in Shorinji Kempo is not to teach the techniques per se but to give nutrition to the heart through Shorinji Kempo. The following six principles, through which I try to achieve the above, are fundamental to the practice of Shorinji Kempo.

1. Kyakkashoko

Kyakkashoko literally means "to take a good look at the area around your feet." It actually refers to the fact that awareness always tends to get ahead of itself. This is all the more so when, for example, you are late. While you are taking your shoes off at the entrance you are thinking of an excuse. Your consciousness is separated from yourself. At least you have enough awareness to arrange your shoes neatly. At that moment, your consciousness returns to yourself. This is kyakkashoko. Do not let your awareness get away from you; keep it at your feet. It is not so much about arranging shoes, rather it is about keeping your awareness and you energy focused on what you are doing at anyone time.

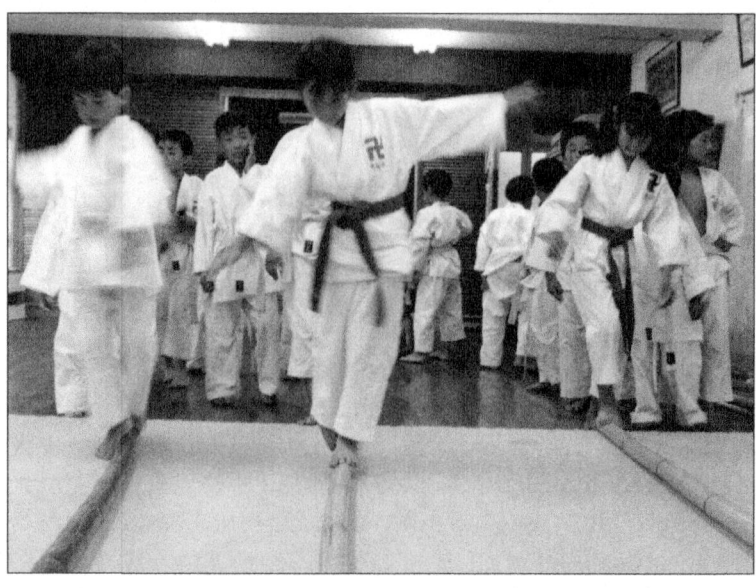

2. Gassho

Gassho is a Buddhist salutation in which you join the palms of your hands together. This gesture symbolizes the unity of mind and body. This unity is important in staying mentally and physically fit and healthy and focused on whatever activity you are doing. Gassho is also a greeting and the purpose of greetings is to get closer to people and to get to know them. Joining the hands together can also be said to symbolize the joining of people to form a harmonious society. It is important to greet people and to get to know people as a whole unified person. Approach each other from the heart.

3. Samu

Samu is the action of cleaning, sweeping, tidying up, and so on. To remove dirt and maintain order in your surroundings cultivates your heart and leads one to remove dirt and disorder from your heart and mind.

4. Chinkongyo

Chinkongyo consists of the recitation of the oaths of Shorinji Kempo and seated meditation. The following principles are important and must be borne in mind when doing chinkongyo: *Choushin* literally means "to bring your body together," thus to straighten your spine. In other words, correct and maintain your posture. *Chousoku*, literally means "bringing your breathing together," to maintain correct breathing. It is interpreted as to find the life force that fills the heaven and earth within one's own body. Choushin is focusing the heart, which enables the whole body to gush forth with energy.

5. Keiko

Keiko literally means "to reflect on past experience" and, therefore, to learn. The term is generally used to mean "to practice." In Shorinji Kempo, keiko is a means to unify one's spirit, energy, and strength. It is a means to find harmony with a partner. It is a way to discover the exquisiteness of an endless supply of techniques and is the source of courage and drive.

6. Howa

Howa are the lectures and discussions about the "way." If the words you speak do not come from the bottom of your heart, they will not reach your opponent's heart. If you open your heart, then your opponent will open his.

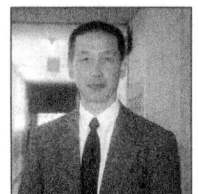
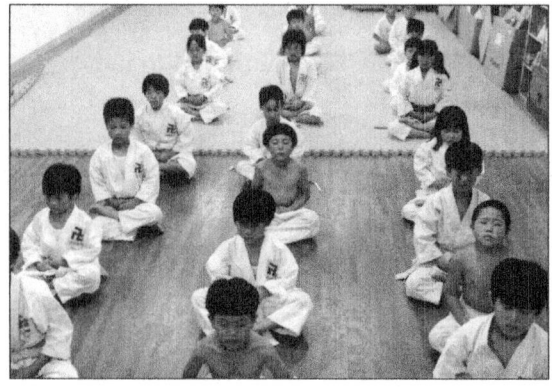

The author, Sakuyama Yoshinaga, and some students.

The founder of Shorinji Kempo, So Doshin, said, "Technique is bait. Your role is to teach how to live as a human being to the people who gather around you because they are attracted by the bait." He taught this to the teachers. Even though he thoroughly understood the feelings of those *kenshi*[3] who are hooked by the exquisiteness of an endless supply of techniques, he still emitted these words. The words came out because he knew clearly what the purpose was.

[3] This could literally be translated as "fist warrior," but it is a standard term in Shorinji Kempo meaning "practitioner."

7. From Kon to Kon Transmission from Teacher to Student

Children's hearts are crying out in desolation, yet no answer can be found. Many people in the world entrust a ray of hope in the martial arts. Now we have seen a post-war limit to education. We can now see the possibilities of the samurai education system as it spanned over several hundred years. They developed the heart through martial culture and martial spirit. However, this possibility does not exist within the competitive ideology. Then again, I cannot believe that those who stress endurance or etiquette have the kon to be able to develop kon in students.

If there is anything that the martial world can achieve in this chaotic educational environment, it will be to transmit through actions from kon to kon the attitude expressed in Dr. Nitobe Inazo's famous work, *Bushido*: "Make oneself into a shining light first" (Buddha). At the very least, it is important that teachers touch the children's hearts with their own heart.

chapter 4

Educating the Mind as Well as the Body Through Martial Arts Training

by Terrence Webster-Doyle, Ph.D.

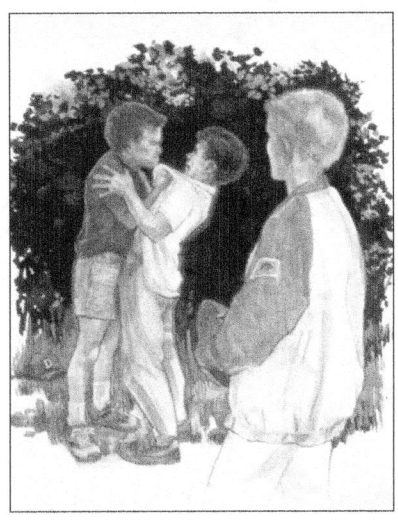

All illustrations courtesy of T. Webster-Doyle.

    We who have been in the martial arts for so many years and love these arts find that there is so much to them. I began studying formally in 1961 (and even earlier via magazines and books), being interested in what seemed to be "mysterious power," the mysticism of the East, a vague and exciting promise of some foreign transcendent experience. This lasted only a short while after months (and years) of hard, grinding, and repetitive work. Thousands of blocks, strikes, punches, and kicks later, I re-evaluated my initial view of the martial arts. But I still had that slightly mysterious feeling deep in my gut that the martial arts were more than just repetitive self-defense techniques. I knew the physical aspects were important, but I felt there was more to it. So I began a serious journey to find out what this more was.

What I found now seems quite obvious, although at the time I thought otherwise. What was hard for me was understanding the "mental" or psychological side of the martial arts. Mostly, the books on martial arts were of two kinds—first it was technique, the "how-to" lessons in self-defense; secondly, it was Eastern philosophy—Daoism, Buddhism, and especially Zen Buddhism with its mind-boggling cryptic stories which left you wondering what you had just read. My Western mind had a difficult time understanding the underlying philosophy of the martial arts because I was looking for "answers," solutions to a problem. It took me years to understand what in essence was quite simple. But that is another story. Suffice it to say that a wonderful haiku poem could encompass the philosophy underlying martial arts practice.

But there was something in this mental side that was "answerable." What the basic intent of the martial arts was telling me was that we study martial arts to end conflict non-violently, not to create more violent conflict. This is what I had felt all along. It was what had attracted me to the martial arts in the first place. It was not what I saw in martial arts movies or magazines. It was not what I saw in many martial arts schools.

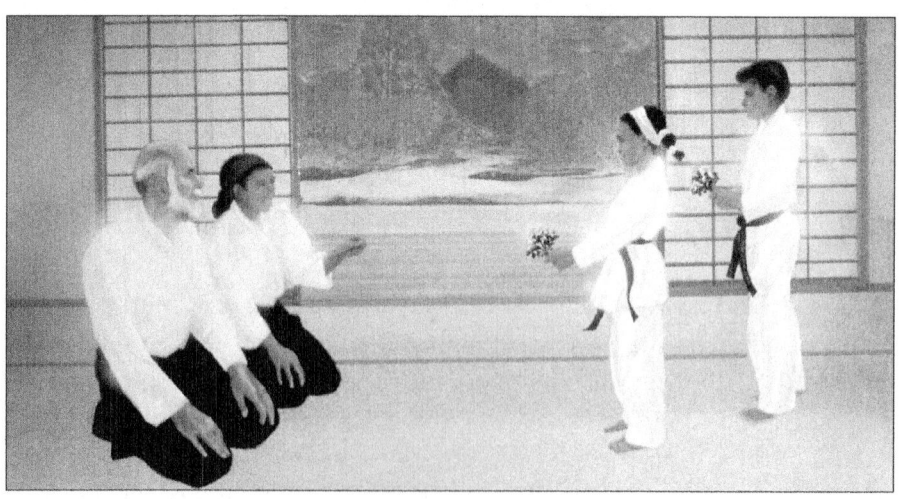

Cultural traditions of the East and West are embedded with educational methods which support peaceful means to end conflict. Can any be recognized in your martial arts classes? Illustration by Rod Cameron.

What I generally saw was martial arts portrayed as bizarre, lethal fighting, a style of conflict resolution through "heroic" violent acts. This was because the basic intent was not understood correctly—that of understanding and ending conflict nonviolently. Most people only saw the physical side—the self-defense portion, and therefore exploited that sensational aspect, removing it from its whole context and meaning. The martial arts therefore became unbalanced, violent in being divided from the whole. I thought about this and decided that in order to carry out the important intent of the martial arts—to end conflict nonviolently —I had to teach more than mere physical self-defense. I had to teach the mental or psychological side—and in a down-to-earth, practical manner—especially when it came to my young students.

There is much I've learned since these initial insights. I have written 21 books on the subject—which is complex, but not overly difficult. I realized the obvious fact that it was vitally important to teach the martial arts in way which included both the physical and the mental—they go together as an integrated whole. One cannot be taught without the other. I realized that physical self-defense skills could give a young person the confidence to not react to a potential threat in a self-defeating fight-or-flight manner.

When one felt this confidence that he or she could handle the situation, a "pause" or "gap" was created in this reaction to threat. What I did then was to give young people the psychological skills to get out of the conflict using nonviolent alternatives; that is, through the use of role-playing they learned how to turn a potentially threatening situation into a peaceful one. Acting out the roles of the bully or the victim, the young people learned how to cope nonviolently with hostility. And, it was so simple and easy!

I realized that this was the first step in creating the right foundation for the mental side of the martial arts. It was a simple, safe, practical and successful way to end conflict without creating more conflict. I found that teaching physical self-defense skills alone wasn't enough. By only teaching the young person to fight, I was removing one of his or her alternatives to a threat—that is, to be able to run away (flight). What I wanted to do was to increase the alternatives so the student could have more options than only the underlying skills of physical self-defense. In most cases, the nonviolent (mental) alternatives worked. The students did not have to rely on self-defense physically. So, I felt that I was putting into practice the original intent of the martial arts—to end conflict peacefully—in a way that any young person could put into practice easily and effectively. The key here was to train my students in these mental skills, just like they were training in the physical skills.

I now see that the martial arts, if taught properly, could help a person understand conflict on all levels, because at the root conflict is conflict—the individual conflict is the world's conflict; both have the same nature and structure in conditioned thinking. But this is another issue that would need to be discussed at length. I now understand that the martial arts can have a vital and profound role in helping people resolve conflict nonviolently. It is clear to me that the martial arts have the potential to become a significant educational model to use in raising young people to be healthy and intelligent human beings. The martial arts can become a vital force in society in changing our conditioned, destructive patterns of relationship and thus, create the potential for a more peaceful and loving world—if they are taught as they were intended to be taught.

chapter 5

Observational Learning in the Martial Art Studio: Instructors as Models of Positive Behaviors

by Anne M.C. Barnfield, Ph.D.

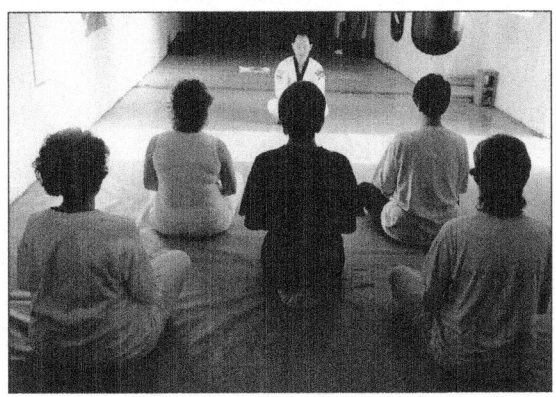

Grandmaster Joon P. Chooi in front of one of his classes
at the Oriental Martial Arts College in Columbus, Ohio.
All photography by Lee Ann McGuire. © 2003

Introduction

That we live in a violent society is a common belief today and each year thousands people are victims of aggression and violence. Aggression has many aspects, including verbal abuse, vandalism, and physical attacks. Thus, even those who have never experienced the intense form, violence, will have encountered aggression in a less intense form, such as verbal insult or hostility. Of increasing concern in our society is aggression by younger persons. Parents are particularly concerned that their children may be victims of violence and are frightened by the thought that there are many opportunities for youngsters to encounter and even learn from aggressive or violent acts performed by others; whether these be face-to-face, real-life experiences or vicarious ones through the media, such as television and, more recently, video games.

Defining Aggression

"Aggression" as a word in everyday use is a broad and very inclusive term, taking in everything from murder to a hurtful remark. For purposes of discussion, it requires more specificity of definition. Bushman and Anderson (2001: 274) wrote that:

> We define human aggression as any behavior directed toward another individual that is carried out with the proximate (immediate) intent to cause harm. In addition, the perpetrator must believe that the behavior will harm the target and that the target is motivated to avoid the behavior.

Thus aggression may be defined as behavior intended to harm or injure another person (either physically or psychologically). Two important implications of this definition are:

1) The goal of the behavior is harm or injury—the keyword being intent, accidental injury is not included.
2) There is an expectation that the behavior will result in harm to the victim. This idea is consistent with that of intent. If a person thinks that their behavior is futile and has no chance of delivering intended harm, that behavior would not be considered aggressive.

Although there may be examples of aggression that do not fit these criteria, these are major points about aggression which cover the majority of cases.

Aggression may be classified into two categories: *instrumental* and *hostile* aggression. Instrumental aggression is designed to achieve a goal or reward beyond aggression itself; e.g. aggression in pursuit of material gain such as assaulting another person during a robbery, fighting in self-defense or in defense of another (prosocial aggression), or to prove one's power or dominance. Hostile (or *affective*) aggression is where the sole aim is to inflict injury and no additional object or motive is involved; e.g., schoolyard bullies. "Affect" is a psychological term meaning having to do with mood, and aggression usually involves negative emotional states (Geen, 1990). Anger is most often thought of as instigating and guiding aggressive behavior. It has been noted, however, that: "the emotional state of anger may be involved in affective aggression *without necessarily causing that aggression*" (Geen, 1990: 5). Even given these definitions, the distinction between hostile and instrumental aggression may not be clear-cut—what looks like hostile aggression may serve other ends.

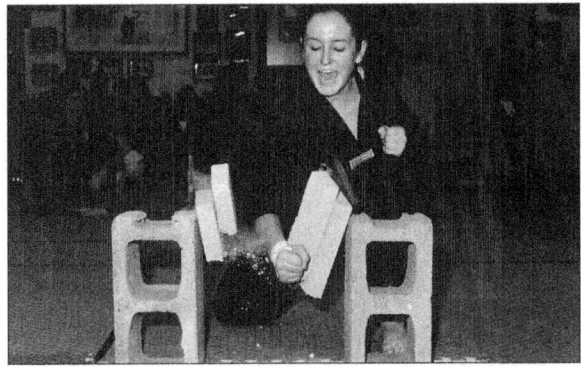

Rachel Kahn testing for her 2nd-degree black belt test at the Oriental Martial Arts College in Columbus, Ohio.

Theoretical Approaches

Because of the pervasiveness of aggression it has been suggested that the will to aggress is a basic instinct. One of the best known theories of innate aggression is the psychoanalytic theory of Sigmund Freud. According to Freud, aggressive instincts are lodged in the unconscious, the deep, least accessible level of mind, and are continuously generated (Freud, 1933/1964). The impulses themselves are kept from consciousness, but influence behavior either outwardly, through overt aggression, or inwardly, in the form of self-destructive acts (Freud, 1933/1964). Freud felt that release of aggressive impulses was necessary, referring to such impulses as *"freely mobile* processes which press towards discharge" (Freud, 1920/1955). This idea is in line with the ancient Greek concept of *catharsis*—a purging of emotion. The tension of the aggressive impulses needed to be released, by aggression against the self or against others (Geen, 1990). If impulses were not released, directly or indirectly, they could overflow into violence. However, there is little direct evidence for this part of the psychoanalytic perspective. Later theorists in the Freudian tradition, such as Dollard and Miller, rejected the idea that aggression was an innate drive or instinct and instead proposed that it was a *frustration produced* drive. Frustration (being thwarted in achieving a goal, for example) could lead to anger, which in turn could lead to aggressive responses (e.g. Dollard, et al, 1939/1961).

Dissatisfaction with the Freudian perspective and development of cognitive and social psychological theories led to alternative explanations regarding aggressive behaviors. In normal individuals, the frequency with which aggressive behavior is expressed, the form it takes, and the situations in which it is displayed are determined largely by learning and by social influences. Psychologists who take a cognitive-social approach usually tend to view aggression as a set of acquired behaviors, and give much less emphasis to the involvement of innate and biological determinants.

Although it has its origins in behaviorism, in which all behavior is explained by stimulus-response conditioning, social learning theory employs a much broader definition and introduces other mechanisms of learning such as imitation and observational learning. These involve some level of cognitive mediation (involvement of thought), which learning theorists would not accept. Contemporary social learning theory thus developed because of what many perceived to be the inadequacies of earlier theories, particularly the traditional learning theory. Previous theories were seen as underemphasizing cognitive variables, being based on animal experimentation, failing to recognize the importance of social and interpersonal forces, and having a view of the human being as a passive recipient of environmental stimulation.

One of the major theorists within the cognitive-social perspective is Albert Bandura. Bandura has stressed that one can learn behaviors vicariously through social models, regardless of rewards or even practice (Bandura, 1969, 1977). For Bandura, people are neither completely autonomous nor do they respond mechanically to environmental influences. They are, instead, active contributors to their own motivation and action. Behavior, thought, emotion, other personal factors and environmental events all combine to determine the individual's actions. Thus personal and environmental factors are interdependent. Frustration may lead to aggression, but the expression of aggression is affected by one's social environment (Bandura and Walters, 1959). One reason that social learning theorists advocate the study of humans in interactions with one another is that each influences the environment and can influence others present. In social learning theory, the process of socialization tends to be seen as a shaping of behavior by external reinforcement, or reward. Behavior is learned in interpersonal situations and linked to the mediation of other people. Most behavior is viewed as being learned, with genetic factors seen as having at best a minor role via an interaction with social reinforcements (Bandura and Walters,

1963). Learning in childhood may be more influential than in adulthood, but adults are not seen as victims of childhood experiences.

Imitation and Observation

With respect to the learning of aggression, there are two major types of learning proposed within social learning theory which have application in explanation of such behavior. *Imitation* and *observation* are key concepts of social learning theory. Much human behavior is learned through observation and imitation. This form of learning can take place without the learner intending to learn or actually being taught. The classic examples of this come from the research Bandura and his colleagues began in the early 1960's (e.g. Bandura, 1969; Bandura, Ross and Ross, 1963; Bandura and Walters, 1963). This research showed that children who watched a model, on television or in real life, will imitate that model's behavior regardless of whether they have been told that imitation will lead to reward. In the now famous "Bobo doll" study, Bandura, Ross and Ross (1963) showed children a film of an adult in a room containing a large clown doll, *Bobo*, and a number of other toys. The adult, while supposedly playing, began to act aggressively toward the doll, punching, kicking and hitting it with other toys. The children were then led into the exact playroom as seen in the film. While the researchers observed from an adjoining room, the children began to act toward Bobo in the same manner as the adults whom they had seen on film. The reproduction of actions was frighteningly exact, with direct imitations of aggressive acts; e.g. hitting, kicking, even throwing the doll. This imitation of aggressive actions is also of concern regarding the increasingly violent video games now available. More recent work has found some similar results in the film and television studies of video games (e.g. Anderson and Dill, 2000; Bartholow and Anderson, 2001) although it has been argued that research regarding such games has shown variable results (Donohue, 2002). Bushman and Anderson (2002), however, argue that the weight of the literature clearly shows that exposure to media violence—including video games—leads to aggressive behavior and that this occurs because exposure to aggression and violence leads to expectations of aggressive responses from others.

Imitation serves to expand the child's repertoire, but in a selective manner with only some aspects of behavior being imitated. There is a difference between learning a behavior and the performance of it. This can be used to distinguish between observational learning and imitation. Bandura and colleagues also showed children a film which depicted adults behaving aggressively toward one another. If the actors were presented as powerful, or rewarded for their behavior, children were more likely to imitate them. If this was not case, the children were less likely to imitate them (Bandura and Walters, 1963). When the researchers offered children rewards specifically for imitating the adults, children who had not previously imitated them did so. These children had learned the behavior, but did not act on it. Thus even if a person attends to and remembers a behavior observed, and has the ability to perform it, they may not actually perform that behavior unless there is sufficient incentive or motivation to do so. Exposure to aggression, even televised aggression, does, though, increase tolerance of real-life aggression (Molitor and Hirsch, 1994; Orobio de Castro, et al, 2002). A meta-analysis by Orobio de Castro et al. (2002), which integrated the results of forty-one studies of aggressive behavior, found that hostile attributions of intent and aggressive reactions were strongly correlated. The greatest effects were found in situations of actual social interaction. Thus as with findings regarding televised or video game violence, viewing of aggressive acts might lead to a concept of aggressive reaction or even of a "first strike" against a perceived aggressive other.

The experiments of Bandura and others have shown that imitation occurs, but perhaps more importantly they have shown that people will perform actions or behaviors after watching *others* being rewarded or punished for doing or not doing those actions. People will do so without receiving any direct reward or punishment themselves, learning by simply watching the behavior with no visible reward attached.

One additional aspect of studies linking the observation of violence to aggression is that the effects seem to be long-lasting. One must exercise caution in interpreting such results, since a correlation, as has been found, does not necessarily explain cause. Although as Eron (1987: 440) stated in the report of his 22-year study on the effects of violence on television: "Early television habits are also related to aggressive behavior 22 years later," it may be that aggressive people watch more television, or more violent programs, not that violence on television causes more aggression. However, as Eron goes on to note: "What was probably important about the programs these children watched were the attitudes and behavioral norms inculcated by watching of those and similar programs. . . . we can consider continued television watching as rehearsal of aggressive sequences" (1987: 440). Similarly, as noted above, one can learn "behavioral norms" by watching aggression in *real-life* situations.

Self-Regulation and Moral Standards

In the basic stimulus-response view of behaviorism, it is external rewards and punishments which are seen as controlling behaviors. If the behavior was rewarded, we will do it again; if not, we try something else. The social learning perspective gives a different view, with the addition of the idea that one should also take into account the possibility of *self-reinforcement*. Social learning theory maintains that much of human behavior is *self-regulated*. In other words, in addition to being governed by external rewards and punishments, our behavior is governed by internal standards. Human thoughts, behaviors, and emotions are influenced by the rewards and punishments we give to ourselves; e.g., pride in achievement, or blame for failure. Consequently, our actions are regulated not only by external reward and punishment, but also by self-regulated standards. These internal standards are learned through rewards and punishments administered by others, and there is evidence to suggest that they can also be acquired on a vicarious basis; e.g. Bandura and Kupers (1964) found that children exposed to models who set high standards reward themselves only for superior performance, while children who observe the behavior of a model who rewards him/herself for low standards may impose lower standards for their own behavior when they perform the same task.

We learn our initial set of internal standards from the behavior of models, typically our parents and other significant people in our life. Once we adopt a standard, we begin a continuous, lifelong process of comparing our behavior to that standard.

Standards of right and wrong, of moral conduct, are also derived from both direct and vicarious experience. As with performance standards, moral principles are usually modelled by the child's parents and other significant adults and are eventually internalized (Bandura, 1969). Once internalized, these moral principles determine which behaviors and thoughts are self-sanctioned and which result in self-contempt. Thus, moral behavior comes to be self-regulated and is maintained independently, and even in spite of, environmental consequences. Bandura (1977: 154) wrote that:

> The anticipation of self-reproach for conduct that violates one's standards provides a source of motivation to keep behavior in line with standards in the face of opposing inducements. There is no more devastating punishment than self-contempt.

Moral behavior also has been linked to aggression. As Cox, Qui and Lui (1993: 19) noted, persons "at a low level of moral reasoning have a difficult time making correct decisions regarding aggression because they do not perceive it as immoral." A higher level of moral reasoning and understanding was seen as necessary to ethical behavior and control of aggression.

In summary, social learning theorists have provided a body of research showing that observational learning takes place in humans. The studies have often focussed on aggressive behavior, one of the major concerns in our society. The conclusions from this research are clear: by merely observing, in real life on television or in films, aggressive behavior that is rewarded (or at least not punished), a person can learn that it pays to be aggressive. This will happen even if the violence is committed by cartoon characters. Such findings raise important questions for a society beset by an increasing rate of violence. In fairness, however, one should note not all portrayals of violence lead to violence in the observer; aggressive behavior may be learned but not performed.

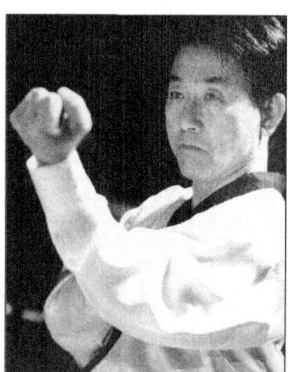 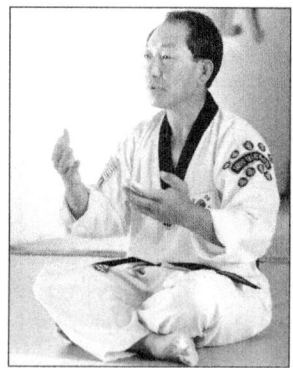

Left: Master Young Choi, head of the Oriental Martial Arts College in Indianapolis, Indiana, practicing. Right: Grandmaster Joon P. Choi sharing the history and philosophy of Asian martial traditions.

Parents worry about children watching aggression in films and on television shows. Research has shown that viewing aggression and violence in the media can influence the subsequent behavior of children, and that viewing of actual models can have the same effect. It would then seem that a parent would have cause to worry about the result of enrolling a child in an activity where aggressive behavior seems the norm: kicking, punching, and other "violent" techniques are taught, and fighting appears to be practiced. The parents may ask themselves, to rephrase the question posed by Kim (1974: 105): "Aren't you turning out killers; aren't you teaching an art that enables violence?" However, as Eron (1987) points out in his report, different responses, behaviors and internalized standards lead a child to act aggressively, or nonaggressively, in a given situation. A child thus needs models of appropriate behavior from whom to learn positive social behaviors. If aggressive models are supplied by the media and by martial arts instructors, and if overly-aggressive behavior is not subject to discipline, the young student will continue to exhibit this type of behavior. Alternatively, observing those who exhibit the opposite behavior, who in the same situation ignore instigation to aggression and remain calm, it is then self-controlled behavior which is imitated (Bandura and Walters, 1963).

Models — Ancient and Modern

In the past, martial arts tended to be regarded more as family secrets, to be passed on to a select few. This led to a more familial-type relationship between the student (who may actually have been the *sensei's* child) and teacher. This aspect of the teacher-student relationship probably led to closer imitation and a greater sense of personal responsibility in the young student, exemplified by Matusumura's words to Sakugawa when presented to the elder martial artist as an aspiring student: "I will not disappoint you" (Kim, 1974: 32). To earlier martial artists, respect was a fundamental principle.

In the modern world, there has been a change in the setting in which martial arts are learned. The common situation now is as a member of a group, all learning at the same time from a *sensei* who may be viewed more as any other teacher is today than as a parental figure or mentor. This attitude may be more extreme in clubs of "sport" styles than in more "traditional" dojos, where the culture is one of respect rather than simple admiration. The *sensei*, in any martial art, in any club or dojo, is the main individual who would definitely be viewed as a model. In the traditional dojo, the watchwords of respect and discipline regulate behavior and appear to lead to an internalization of positive self-standards.

Time and again, the writings of the masters show concern with "right behavior" and moral conduct, not with aggressive responses, despite the unsettled or even warlike times in which they may have lived. Examples from earlier times may be found in the translation of the *Bubishi* by McCarthy (1995): "disciples must pledge to never intentionally hurt anyone or do anything unjust" (p. 68). "The true meaning of [martial arts] lies not in victory or defeat, but rather, in patience, sincerity, honesty, and benevolence" (p. 69). "True *quanfa* disciples never seek to harm anyone, but are virtuous, kind, and responsible human beings" (p. 91). In more recent history, Funakoshi Ginchin (1869-1957), writing in his autobiography *Karate-do, My Way of Life* (1956/1975: 104), stated that:

> he who thinks of himself alone and is inconsiderate of others is not qualified to learn Karate-do. . . . Nonetheless, there are always some whose only desire is to learn karate so as to make use of it in a fight. These almost inevitably drop out of the course before half a year has passed, for it is quite impossible for any young person whose objective is so foolish to continue very long at karate.

There is no doubt that Master Funakoshi thought the learning of karate for aggressive purposes was wrong, a "foolish" notion. A view reinforced in his famous maxim: "In karate there is no first attack" ("In karate, one does not make the first move"; Kim, 1982: 98).

Regarding aggression, the important aspect of modelling by the traditional sensei is that aggression is seen as a controlled act, within a particular situation and for a certain purpose—it is not an end in itself (hostile aggression), nor should raw aggression be a means to an end (instrumental aggression). As Kim wrote, in answering his own question rephrased above: "there is a morality involved, woven in the fabric of karate, that controls the violence and the use of the art except under one condition—absolute necessity and dire peril" (1974: 105).

Although it has been argued that there is only "tentative support for the notion that the discipline of the martial arts may reduce assaultive hostility rather than serve as a model for such behavior" (Daniels and Thornton, 1990: 95), a number of studies have shown that aggressiveness (by several measures) actually *declines* with increase in years training and rank in a variety of martial arts (e.g. Lamarre and Nosanchuck, 1999; Nosanchuck, 1981; Skelton, Glynn and Berta, 1991). In an intriguing study, Trulson (1986) showed that instruction in a traditional martial arts style (Tae Kwon Do) actually improved behavior of juvenile delinquents. In this study, three groups of delinquents were given traditional-style training, "modern" style training, or physical activities in a gym. The modern style and general activities improved physical fitness, but neither had positive effects on behavior; in fact, students trained in the modern style "showed an even greater tendency toward delinquency . . . than they did at the beginning of the study" (Trulson, 1986: 1131). In contrast, the traditional training style led not only to physical improvement, but also to behavioral improvement in those assigned to that group, including a decline in aggressiveness (Trulson, 1986). A survey comparison of students from traditional versus modern dojos by Nosanchuck and MacNeil (1989) provides support for Trulson's (1986) findings and notes that the effect was due to *training* rather than self-selection. Students who continued training in a traditional style ("stayers") showed a decline in aggressiveness with belt level, apparently as a result of learning. It was not that the more aggressive persons dropped out, leaving a dojo of only the naturally less aggressive, but that reduction in aggression occurred due to a training style "where students are socialized into aggression control" (Nosanchuck and MacNeil, 1989: 158).

One additional aspect of modelling to note is the influence of the sex of the model. Bandura and colleagues' work, as mentioned above (e.g. Bandura, 1969; Bandura and Walters, 1963), showed the aspects of the model which are important in encouraging imitation, such as status, reward, and also if the model were the same sex as the observers. Therefore an important factor in the modern dojo may be the presence of female models, both as senior students and instructors. These women martial artists not only counter sex-stereotyping for all students, but also provide same-sex models for younger female students, a type of student probably more common in modern dojos than in those of historical times.

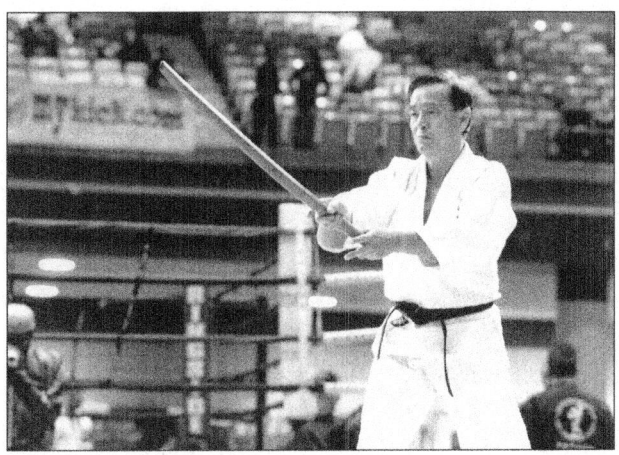

Swordsman Seiji Tanaka maneuvering with precision
during an exhibition at the Battle of Columbus.

Conclusions

Is a person learning karate, an apparently aggressive practice, going to become increasingly aggressive and violent? From the theory and research presented here the answer to this question is "no," but it is a qualified no. Children especially are impressionable and "easily led," but this will not be a problem if the right model is provided. Here then is the qualifier to the answer; it is the appropriateness of the model which is key. What is needed, as stated in the motto of Legacy Shorin Ryu Karate, is *"traditional karate for modern times."* If an individual is practicing a traditional style martial art, where respect and discipline are paramount, with a knowledgeable and caring instructor—a true *sensei*—what is learned will be far from violence. The student will have a proper model, and will grow in body, mind, and spirit.

BIBLIOGRAPHY

ANDERSON, C. AND DILL, K. (2000). Video games and aggressive thoughts, feelings and behavior in the laboratory and in life. *Journal of Personality and Social Psychology, 78*(4), 772-790.

BANDURA, A. (1969). *Principles of behavior modification*. New York: Holt, Rinehart and Winston.

BANDURA, A. (1977). *Social learning theory*. Englewood Cliffs, NJ: Prentice Hall.

BANDURA, A. and KUPERS, C. (1964). Transmission of patterns of self-reinforcement through modelling. *Journal of Abnormal and Social Psychology, 69*, 1-9.

BANDURA, A., ROSS, D., AND ROSS, S. (1963). Imitation of film-mediated aggressive models. *Journal of Abnormal and Social Psychology, 66*(1), 3-11.

BANDURA, A. and WALTERS, R. (1959). *Adolescent aggression*. New York: Ronald Press.

BANDURA, A. and WALTERS, R. (1963). *Social learning and personality development*. New York: Holt Reinhart Publishers.

BARTHOLOW, B. AND ANDERSON, C. (2002). Effects of violent video games on aggressive behavior: Potential sex differences. *Journal of Experimental Social Psychology, 39*, 283-290.

BUSHMAN, B. AND ANDERSON, C. (2002). Violent video games and hostile expectations: A test of the general aggression model. *Personality and Social Psychology Bulletin, 28*, 1679-1686.

DANIELS, K. AND THORTON, E. (1990). An analysis of the relationship between hostility and training in the martial arts. *Journal of Sports*

Sciences, 8, 95-101.

DOLLARD, J., DOOB, L., MILLER, N., MOWRER, O., AND SEARS, R. (1961). *Frustration and aggression*. New Haven, CT: Yale University Press. (Original work published 1939).

DONOHUE, J. (2002). Virtual enlightenment: The martial arts, cyberspace, and American culture. *Journal of Asian Martial Arts, 11*(2), 8-27.

ERON, L. (1987). The development of aggressive behavior from the perspective of a developing behaviorism. *American Psychologist, 42*(5), 435-442.

FREUD, S. (1964). Beyond the pleasure principle. In J. Strachey (Ed. and Trans.), *The standard edition of the complete psychological works of Sigmund Freud* (Vol. 18, pp. 7-64). London: Hogarth Press. (Original work published 1920).

FREUD, S. (1964). New introductory lectures on psycho-analysis. In J. Strachey (Ed. and Trans.), *The standard edition of the complete psychological works of Sigmund Freud* (Vol. 22, pp. 7-182). London: Hogarth Press. (Original work published 1933).

FREUD, S. (1964). Why war? In J. Strachey (Ed. and Trans.), *The standard edition of the complete psychological works of Sigmund Freud* (Vol. 22, pp. 199-215). London: Hogarth Press. (Original work published 1933).

FUNAKOSHI, G. (1956/1975). *Karate-do—My way of life*. New York: Kodansha.

GEEN, R. (1990). *Human aggression*. Pacific Grove, CA: Brooks/Cole Publishing.

KIM, R. (1974). *The weaponless warriors*. Santa Clarita, CA: Ohara Publications.

KIM, R. (1984). *The classical man*. Hamilton, ON: Masters Publication.

LAMARRE, B. AND NOSANCHUCK, T. (1999). Judo–the gentle way: A replication of studies on martial arts and aggression. *Perceptual and Motor Skills, 88*, 992-997.

MCCARTHY, P. (1985). *The bible of karate: Bubishi*. North Clarendon, VT: Tuttle.

MOLITOR, F. AND HIRSCH, K. (1994). Children's toleration of real-life aggression after exposure to media violence: A replication of the Drabman and Thomas studies. *Child Study Journal, 24*(3), 191-207.

NOSANCHUCK, T. (1981). The way of the warrior: The effects of traditional martial arts training on aggressiveness. *Human Relations, 34*(6), 435-444.

NOSANCHUCK, T. AND MACNEIL, M. (1989). Examination of the effects of traditional and modern martial arts training on aggressiveness. *Aggressive Behavior*, 15, 153-159.

OROBIO DE CASTRO, B., VEERMAN, J., KOOPS, W., BOSCH, J., AND MONSHOUWER, H. (2002). Hostile attribution of intent and aggressive behavior: A metaanalysis. *Child Development*, 73(3), 916-934.

SKELTON, D., GLYNN, M., AND BERTA, S. (1991). Aggressive behavior as a function of taekwondo ranking. *Perceptual and Motor Skills*, 72, 179-182.

Trulson, M. (1986). Martial arts training: a novel "cure" for juvenile delinquency. *Human Relations*, 39(12), 1131-1140.

chapter 6

Information and Strategies for Martial Arts Instructors Working with Children Diagnosed with AttentionDeficit/Hyperactivity Disorder

by Eric K. Cooper, Ph.D.

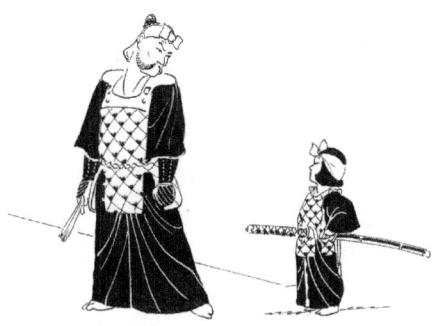

All illustrations from *Tales of the Hermit Vol. III* by O. Ratti and A. Westbrook, published by Via Media Publishing Company. ©2004 by Futuro Designs and Publications.

Attention-Deficit/Hyperactivity Disorder in the Martial Arts

It seems that everywhere we turn today, including television advertisements, newspaper headlines, and magazine and book titles, the letters ADD and ADHD are prominent. Misconceptions abound regarding Attention-deficit Disorder and Attention-deficit/hyperactivity Disorder. Many readers may assume ADHD is the result of poor parenting. Others may believe there is a biological cause for the disorder. Some may not know of the disorder and still others may have preconceived notions and biases. Regardless, children with ADHD are enrolling in martial arts classes across the country, and martial arts instructors may not be familiar with the disorder and may need education concerning ADHD. There are several reasons martial arts instructors should understand ADHD, its causes, symptoms, and how best to address children and parents facing it. Knowing more about ADHD can help a martial arts instructor understand children with ADHD better, help the instructor work better with them, insure that issues of confidentiality are adhered to, and help plan a program of study best suited for each child. The purpose of this chapter is to familiarize martial arts instructors with ADHD, offer current research concerning the benefits of martial arts training for children with ADHD, provide information regarding issues of confidentiality for students with ADHD, and to present additional strategies for working with children with this disorder.

Attention-Deficit/Hyperactivity Disorder

There are many misconceptions and misunderstandings about ADHD. This section will help educate and familiarize the reader with appropriate terminology, symptoms, and current prevalence rates. Please note that person first language (saying and stating that a child has ADHD, not that the child is an ADHD child) is used throughout this chapter and is appropriate and preferred when working with students with ADHD. Remember, these students have ADHD, but this disorder does not define who they are.

According to the *Diagnostic and Statistical Manual* (DSMIV-TR, 2000) of the American Psychiatric Association, the primary diagnostic tool of psychologists in the United States, Attention-Deficit/Hyperactivity Disorder is defined as "a persistent pattern of inattention and/or hyperactivity-impulsivity that is more frequently displayed and more severe than is typically observed in individuals at a comparable level of development" (p. 85). The DSM-IV-TR states that somewhere between 3-7% of school-aged children have ADHD. Common symptoms of ADHD include inattention, impulsivity, hyperactivity, and sometimes aggression, which was one of the symptoms I focused on in my research (Cooper, 2005a). In the past, it was thought that children outgrow the symptoms of ADHD; however, researchers now believe that children do not grow out of ADHD (Barkley, 1996; Joughin, Ramchandant, Zwi, 2003) and that as many as one-third of these children will continue with these symptoms into adulthood (Swanson et al., 1998).

It is important to note that according to the DSM-IV-TR (2000), ADHD is the correct terminology regardless of whether a child is primarily hyperactive or inattentive. Interestingly enough, the outdated terminology, Attention-Deficit Disorder (ADD), seems now to be reserved in popular media for adults with attention problems. Predominately, but in no way exclusionary, boys with ADHD exhibit symptoms of hyperactivity while girls with ADHD exhibit symptoms of inattention.

Each set of symptoms offers its own challenges. However, it also should be noted that each child will exhibit unique symptoms and working with one child with ADHD will probably require different techniques than working with another child with ADHD. It is important to understand that just because a person has had experience with one or two children with ADHD does not mean that person has experienced all the unique combinations of ADHD symptoms that are possible.

Children who exhibit hyperactive behaviors offer different challenges than do those who exhibit inattentive behaviors. Children with hyperactivity often exhibit the following symptoms: fidgeting, running, squirming, and energetic playing (DSM-IV-TR, 2000). Remember, these are behaviors in the extreme and are more pronounced than in typical play and behavior. In addition, hyperactive symptoms are more noticeable and often require constant attention from parents, teachers, and instructors. Whereas, children who exhibit inattentive behaviors, which include the inability to attend, or 'pay attention', to tasks and details (DSM-IV-TR), are often overlooked because they do not require constant monitoring. Unfortunately, this can be detrimental to the inattentive child. An inattentive child may be perceived as paying attention, when in fact, the child is not paying attention and is not learning the offered material. Therefore, children with Attention-Deficit/Hyperactivity Disorder, Predominately Inattentive Type, which tends to be girls, are often overlooked and are missing the help and guidance afforded to children with Predominately Hyperactive Type.

Most diagnoses of ADHD will be of either Predominately Hyperactive Type or Predominately Inattentive Type. However, there is another diagnosis, Combined Type, in which children exhibit both symptoms. Another important issue for instructors to understand is that many children with ADHD, estimates of up to 50% (DSM-IV-TR, 2000; Pliszka, 2003), also are diagnosed with another childhood disorder, such as conduct disorder, oppositional defiant disorder, or learning disabilities. This further complicates diagnoses and highlights the uniqueness of each child.

Research on the Effects of Martial Arts for Children with ADHD

Many popular media sources, including *Parenting a Child with Attention Deficit/Hyperactivity Disorder* (Boyles and Contadino, 1997), *ADD/ADHD Behavior-Change Resource Kit* (Flick, 1998), *Understanding ADHD* (Green and Chee, 1998) and *ADD and the College Student* (Quinn, 2001), suggest that martial arts training is an appropriate intervention, or at least an additional component of a comprehensive treatment program, for children with ADHD. Unfortunately, much of the evidence supporting the use of the martial arts as an intervention for ADHD is anecdotal; much of this support comes from individual cases with little or no supporting research. There has been a serious lack of empirical evidence to support these suggestions. Fortunately, three doctoral studies have been completed to help support these findings.

First Study

Felmet (1998) conducted the first of these doctoral studies with boys diagnosed with ADHD. Felmet paired twenty sets of boys to determine the effects of eight weeks of martial arts training on symptoms of ADHD. Using the Gordon Diagnostic System and the Attention-Deficit Disorders Evaluation Scale, Felmet measured post-test scores in the levels of delay, vigilance, distractibility, inattentiveness, and hyperactive-impulsivity. Felmet postulated eleven hypotheses in her study, and while only two were supported statistically, the results of nine of the hypotheses indicated scores suggesting that the martial arts involvement may have had some positive impact on ADHD.

Although Felmet's (1998) research involved the largest number of participants of the three studies, she also relied on statistical significance. Felmet initially began the study with a total of 40 boys, but ended the study with only 34 participants. This loss of six participants may have contributed to the deficiency of statistical significance. Unfortunately, as many of us in the martial arts know, retention of students at the early levels is increasingly difficult as parents become more savvy consumers and we begin to vie for students' attention with video games and other sports. I ran across such hurdles in my own research, having one potential young participant opt not to begin the study because the taekwondo looked "too hard," while another young participant did not begin because his mother stated she "couldn't get him away from his video games."

Second Study

The second dissertation study, conducted by Morand (2004), investigated the influence of martial arts participation on academic performance as indicated by assessment of homework completion, classroom rules adherence, task redirection, and impulsive actions in the classroom. Whereas Felmet's (1998) research was centered on analysis of task completion and attention duration, Morand's study focused more on the analysis of classroom related behaviors. Morand studied eighteen boys ages 8-11 with ADHD who were divided into three groups: martial arts group, exercise group, and control group.

Morand's results suggested that both the martial arts group and the exercise group were positively influenced by the experience. It is not surprising that the exercise group was impacted as research has been conducted in this area (Etscheidt and Ayllon, 1987; Klein and Deffenbacher, 1977; Tantillo, Kesick, Hynd, and Dishman, 2002) and suggests that an exercise program can positively affect children with ADHD. Although exercise programs have been supported, martial arts programs have had little empirical backing, and Morand's study aimed to support martial arts as a superior treatment program to that of exercise alone. Although Morand summarizes in his study that the martial arts intervention program was more positive in the study than the exercise intervention, a more detailed analysis should be examined by hypothesis in his dissertation.

Third Study

Although Felmet's (1998) results were not supported by statistical significance, her results indicated the possibility of practical significance. The term practical significance, typically used in applied research, suggests the outcome may provide improvement for the subject, family, or situation, but could not be supported statistically (Hersen and Barlow, 1976). For example, a child's symptoms of hyperactivity may decrease only slightly but have a significant improvement in levels of punishment or attention. The study I conducted (Cooper, 2005a) supplemented Felmet's study and used a research design emphasizing practical significance.

I assessed inattention, hyperactivity, impulsivity, and aggression in six children for seven weeks before any martial arts training and then during twelve weeks of taekwondo training to determine treatment results. My results indicated a mixed effect, but results tended toward the positive. The following is a brief description of my research.

The design used for the study was the single-subject design, which is often used by clinicians to determine the outcomes of interventions when the numbers of participants in the study are limited. This design uses participants as their own controls by establishing a baseline of current levels of the behaviors before the intervention, introducing the intervention, and then continuing to assess the participants' behaviors during the intervention to determine the effects of the intervention.

Taekwondo was the martial arts style used as the intervention in this study based on my access to the style and the data that suggests taekwondo is the most popular style of martial arts in the United States (Corcoran, J., and Graden, J, 2001; Lawler, 2003). The participants of the study included five boys and one girl between the ages of six and eleven.

The average age of the participants was approximately eight years of age, and all participants were officially diagnosed with ADHD. Other diagnoses, such as Oppositional Defiant Disorder, Asperger's Syndrome, Dyslexia, and an anxiety disorder, also were present in some of the participants.

During the course of the study, participants were continually assessed by three sources: parents, independent observers, and school teachers. Parents and independent observers completed the ADHD rating scales and an aggression instrument every two weeks during the baseline and the intervention phases. School teachers completed the instruments before and after the intervention to create post-test / pre-test results for additional information.

The results of this study are encouraging for parents of children with ADHD. Four of the six participants showed positive changes in many of the symptoms (inattention, impulsivity, and hyperactivity) associated with ADHD. There were no increases of aggression in the school and only one participant showed any increase in aggression in the home environment (one participant decided to try some kicks on the family dog). In addition, the researcher tracked the ADHD Index Scores (the scores that offer an overall evaluation of the severity of ADHD) of each participant, and results of the index indicate overall positive changes for a majority of the participants.

Based on the results of these three studies, there is reason to further investigate the nature of the martial arts as an intervention for children with ADHD. Several changes to the studies are suggested, including the need for larger sample sizes, changes in martial arts styles and instructors, more control groups, and increases in the number of female participants. Additional areas of research and/or changes in methodology will help to paint a much clearer picture of the use of the martial arts for children with ADHD. With cautious optimism, there is cause to believe that the martial arts may indeed be used as part of a comprehensive treatment plan for ADHD. However, treatment should be monitored continually to ensure the intervention is having the desired effects.

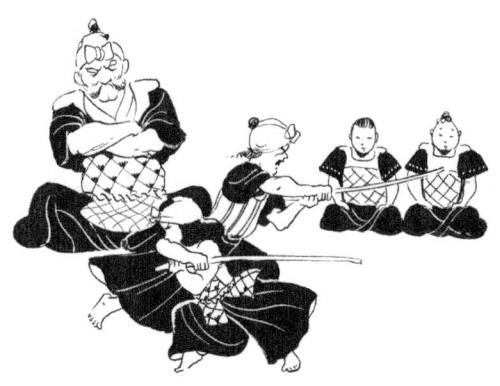

Confidentiality

Of primary concern in the field of psychology is the issue of confidentiality. This is especially true when dealing with diagnosed psychological disorders. Although many parents will be vocal about their children's ADHD diagnosis, and will be the consummate advocates for rights to educational support and funding in the school systems, others are not as vocal and may wish to keep an ADHD diagnosis quiet. In fact, parents typically vocal in the public school system may wish to keep a diagnosis under wraps in other situations, including the martial arts school. The hesitation of parents to publicly announce an ADHD diagnosis may be due to the fact that many people consider ADHD to be caused by bad parenting or that no such condition exists in the first place. Although there is ample evidence to support that ADHD is caused by a biological condition (Maayan et al., 2003; Pary, Lewis, Matuschka, and Lippmann, 2002; Stubberfield, Wray, and Parry, 1999), the fact that many children are misdiagnosed, and overly diagnosed in many instances, perhaps contributes to these misconceptions.

Regardless of the reason, parents and their children have a right to privacy and confidentiality. Parents may bring their children to martial arts classes to ease the symptoms associated with ADHD, including self-esteem issues (Ashley, 2005), and they may even confide in the instructor that their children have ADHD. However, this sharing of information with the instructor does not mean the diagnosis is now public knowledge. It is important that instructors remember not to share sensitive information with others. Although a diagnosis of ADHD may not appear to be sensitive information to one person, it may be extremely so to another. I would even suggest an instructor gain permission from parents to discuss a child's diagnosis with assistant instructors if such discussion is deemed necessary. In addition, some instructors who have had particular success in working with children with ADHD may wish to advertise this fact, using testimonials of parents who may potentially be a reference for that success. Again, the instructor should discuss this intention with these parents to insure public disclosure is appropriate and not unwanted.

I cannot stress enough the importance of confidentiality when it comes to discussing officially diagnosed disorders. I would even go so far as to say that in today's litigious society, a slip of the tongue regarding a protected disorder might be just as detrimental to a martial arts school as physical injury has been in the past. Legal action notwithstanding, upset parents can be damaging to an instructor's reputation and marketability. So, when in doubt, do not mention any disorders that students may have.

Strategies for Working with Children with ADHD

To say that most people have heard of ADHD is probably not much of a stretch. However, many people probably have not worked directly with children with ADHD, or if they have, they may not have recognized the situation. Now, as more students are being diagnosed with ADHD and parents are trying to find ways to relieve the symptoms, more of these children are becoming our students. So, how do we train martial artists, which include instructors and assistant instructors, to work with these children? What are the best practices or best tips when working with a student with ADHD? This section will hopefully offer some helpful tips when working with children with ADHD. As a word of caution, remember that each child with ADHD is a unique individual. One strategy may work with one child, but not another. One child may respond in a positive manner while another may react completely different. It will be necessary for each instructor to determine which strategies work best for which child in his or her school.

There are many books that offer suggestions to parents and teachers on how to work best with children with ADHD, and I would suggest you look to these books for guidance (figure 1). In addition, there also are some publications that offer specific suggestions for working with difficult children in the martial arts or other exercise programs (figure 2). These references can be invaluable in helping martial arts instructors determine the best strategies for dealing with children with ADHD that are appropriate to use with their teaching style or the atmosphere of the training hall that they have created. Unfortunately, these resources, and the suggestions I list next, may require the martial arts instructor to change his or her teaching style, strategies, or the atmosphere of the training hall. Each person must first decide if that can be accomplished.

The following is a list of helpful strategies and tips from the resources offered in the readings lists as applied to the martial arts that can be used with children with ADHD. Please remember that a strategy that works with one child may not work with another, and it may be necessary to make a very realistic and truthful review of your training method, assistant instructors, and actions.

- *Be consistent* – in your actions, comments, expectations, rewards, and disciplinary actions so that children understand what is expected every time.

- *Understand time requirements* – a 90-minute class will probably not be effective for children with ADHD. Neither may an hour class. Certain students may need to be limited to 30 or 45 minutes.

- *Vary your teaching techniques* – although it is important to be consistent in your behaviors and expectations, it also is important to vary the exercises in class. This novelty, which catches the child's attention, helps the child with ADHD pay attention (Sher, 2006). However, be clear in the process for change and how children are expected to move from one activity to the other.

- *Be clear in your directions and use students' names* – capture your students' attention by using their names and hold their attention by using direct language.

- *Set clear and concise rules* – let the child know exactly what the rules are, and be consistent when implementing the rules. Say what you mean and mean what you say so as not to confuse the issue.

- *Learn to use positive reinforcement* – if you use an overabundance of punishment in class, learn to vary your methods and reward good behavior. Positive attention and rewards are a must.

- *Require desirable behaviors* – it is not enough to punish undesirable behaviors. A good teacher will indicate the desired behavior or reframe how a student should behave. Never assume a child with ADHD understands why a behavior is not appropriate. In education, we call this a 'teachable moment'.

- *Check the structure of your classes* – make sure your children with ADHD can see and follow appropriate role models. Do not put a child with ADHD directly with a child who misbehaves or performs techniques inadequately.

- *Set reasonable goals and challenges* – it is important to allow a child with ADHD to succeed. Set individual and reasonable goals for each class. Remember, these children have trouble concentrating and following directions, and may require simple commands. They may need more time to understand or master specific tasks.

- *Understand the effect of competitiveness on the child* – understand whether competition will help the child or encourage the child to misbehave.

There are two other articles readers also may find helpful as resources. The first, "Using Observational Learning Methods for Martial Arts Teaching and Training" (Cooper, 2005b), was inspired by working with young children and other children with attentional problems. This information can be used to determine the visual and auditory set-up and nature of the training hall and help better understand the nature of how children learn merely by watching other students. My article should help an instructor understand how information can be grouped or broken down into easily understood information, how self-talk can be important for a child with ADHD, and other areas or processes that affect learning.

An additional source of information for ADHD and martial arts is *Teaching Difficult Children* by Kim (1999). He devotes much of this publication to working with children with ADHD. Unfortunately, some of the academic information is inaccurate and other parts are now out of date, but the sections highlighting strategies to use with these children are solid and should be considered. Some excellent ideas from Kim's publication include:

- Offering ideas for class structure;
- Modeling appropriate behaviors;
- Giving specific action messages that are clear;
- Using positive reinforcement;
- Replacing undesirable behaviors with desirable behaviors;
- Using time-out systems;

- Making punishments appropriate; and
- Providing immediate feedback.

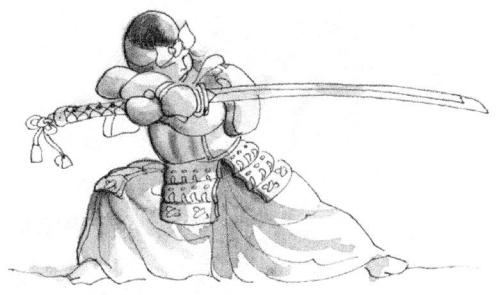

Conclusion

The diagnosis of Attention-deficit/Hyperactivity Disorder is recognized in more children today than five or ten years ago. More of these children are finding their way into martial arts classes as parents are searching for ways to help their children deal with the symptoms associated with this disorder. As this trend continues, it is necessary for martial arts teachers and instructors to understand this disorder and how these children are affected by it and how in turn these children then affect our training halls and schools. It is to be hoped that this chapter has offered helpful information concerning Attention-deficit/Hyperactivity disorder, the symptoms associated with it, and proper terminology and sensitivity. Also, it is necessary for everyone to understand that each child with ADHD is unique. Although many people stereotype children with ADHD as either hyper or lacking attention, the disorder is much more complex than those ideas convey and varying levels of hyperactivity, impulsivity, and inattention combine to create unique and varied individuals.

Current research concerning martial arts as an intervention for ADHD has been offered in hopes that other researchers will see the need for continued study in this area and will work to create programs that can be evaluated for their effectiveness with ADHD. There is no miracle cure for ADHD. Continued research into this disorder may offer additional information concerning the effectiveness of exercise and the martial arts for children with ADHD, but it is important to understand that instructor characteristics and teaching methods are an important influence on any possible benefits offered by the martial arts. I hope that after reading the section on confidentiality instructors now realize the importance of keeping information in confidence so as to cause no harm, even inadvertently, to their students or their families.

I also hope the tips and strategies, however briefly offered, for working with children with ADHD will help instructors when dealing with students in their training halls. The suggestions for further reading listed in figures 1 and 2 can give more detailed information that may be tailored for each individual student. My desire is that parents and families will bring more of their children into our training facilities, provided the children enjoy the experience, in hopes of alleviating the symptoms associated with ADHD.

Figure 1
List of General Books on ADHD

Alexander-Roberts, C. (2006). *The AD/HD parenting handbook*. Boulder, CO: Taylor Trade.

Ashley, S. (2005). *The ADD & ADHD answer book*. Naperville, IL: Sourcebooks.

Barkley, R. A. (2000). *Taking charge of ADHD*. New York: Guilford Press.

Green, C. and Chee, K. (1997). *Understanding ADHD*. London, UK: Vermillion.

Lawlis, F. (2005). *The ADD answer: How to help your child now*. New York: Plume Books.

Figure 2
List of Exercise and Martial Arts Related Books and Articles

Kim, S. H. (1999). *Teaching difficult children*. Wethersfield, CT: Turtle Press.

Putnam, S. (2001). *Nature's ritalin for the marathon mind: Nurturing your ADHD child with exercise*. Hinesberg, VT: Upper Access.

Sher, B. (2006). *Attention games*. Hoboken, NJ: John Wiley and Sons.

REFERENCES

AMERICAN PSYCHIATRIC ASSOCIATION. (2000). *Diagnostic and statistical manual of mental disorders.* Washington, DC: American Psychiatric Association.

ASHLEY, S. (2005). *The ADD and ADHD answer book.* Naperville, IL: Sourcebooks.

BARKLEY, R. (1996). Attention-deficit hyperactivity disorder. In E. J. Mash and R. A. Barkley (Eds.), *Child psychopathology* (pp. 63-112). New York, NY: Guilford Press.

COOPER, E. (2005a). The effects of martial arts on inattention, impulsivity, hyperactivity, and aggression in children with attention-deficit/hyperactivity disorder: A single-subject multiple-baseline design across participants. Unpublished doctoral dissertation, Capella University, Minnesota.

COOPER, E. (2005b). Using observational learning methods for martial arts teaching and training. *Journal of Asian Martial Arts, 14*(3), 8-21.

CORCORAN, J., AND GRADEN, J. (2001). *The ultimate martial arts Q&A book.* Chicago, IL: Contemporary Books.

ETSCHEIDT, M., AND AYLLON, T. (1987). Contingent exercise to decrease hyperactivity. *Journal of Child and Adolescent Psychotherapy, 4,* 192-198.

FELMET, M. (1998). The effects of karate training on the levels of attention and impulsivity of children with attention deficit/hyperactivity disorder. Unpublished doctoral dissertation, The University of Toledo, Ohio.

HERSEN, M., AND BARLOW, D. (1976). *Single-case experimental designs: Strategies for studying behavior change.* New York, NY: Pergamon Press.

JOUGHIN, C., RAMCHANDANT, P., AND ZWI, M. (2003). Attention-deficit/hyperactivity disorder. *American Family Physician, 67,* 1969-1970.

KIM, S.H. (1999). *Teaching difficult children.* Wethersfield, CT: Turtle Press.

KLEIN, S., AND DEFFENBACHER, J. (1977). Relaxation and exercise for hyperactive impulsive children. *Perceptual and Motor Skills, 45,* 1159-1162.

LAWLER, J. (2003). *Martial arts for dummies.* New York, NY: Wiley Publishing.

MAAYAN, R., YORAN-HEGESH, R., STROUS, R., NECHMAD, A., AVERBUCH, E., WEIZMAN, A., AND SPIVAK, B. (2003). Three-month treatment course of methylphenidate increases plasma levels of dehydroepiandrosterone (DHEA) and dehydroepiandrosterone-sulfate (DHEA-S) in attention deficit hyperactivity disorder. *Neuropsychobiology, 48,* 111-115.

MORAND, M. (2004). The effects of mixed martial arts and exercise on behavior of boys with attention deficit hyperactivity disorder. Unpublished doctoral dissertation, Hofstra University, New York.

PARY, R., LEWIS, S., MATUSCHKA, P. R., AND LIPPMANN, S. (2002). Attention-deficit/hyperactivity disorder: An update. *Southern Medical Journal*, 95, 743-749.

PLISZKA, S. (2003). Psychiatric comorbidities in children with attention deficit hyperactivity disorder: Implications for management. *Pediatric Drugs*, 5, 741-750.

SHER, B. (2006). *Attention games*. San Francisco, CA: Jossey-Bass.

STUBBERFIELD, T., WRAY, J., AND PARRY, T. (1999). Utilization of alternative therapies in attention-deficit hyperactivity disorder. *Journal of Pediatric Child Health*, 35, 450-453.

SWANSON, J., SERGEANT, J, TAYLOR, E., SONUGA-BARKE, E., JENSEN, P., AND CANTWELL, D. (1998). Attention-deficit hyperactivity disorder and hyperkinetic disorder. *Lancet*, 351, 429-433.

TANTILLO, M., KESICK, C., HYND, G, AND DISHMAN, R. (2002). The effects of exercise on children with attention-deficit hyperactivity disorder. *Medicine and Science in Sports and Exercise*, 34(2), 203-212.

chapter 7

Reflections on an After-School Literacy Program and the Educational Value of Taekwondo: A Preliminary Analysis

by Derek Van Rheenen, Ph.D.

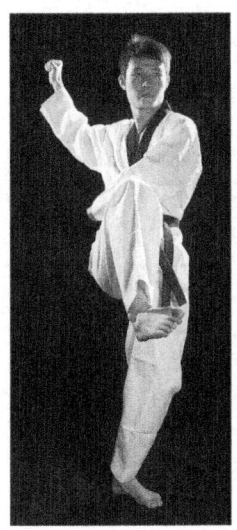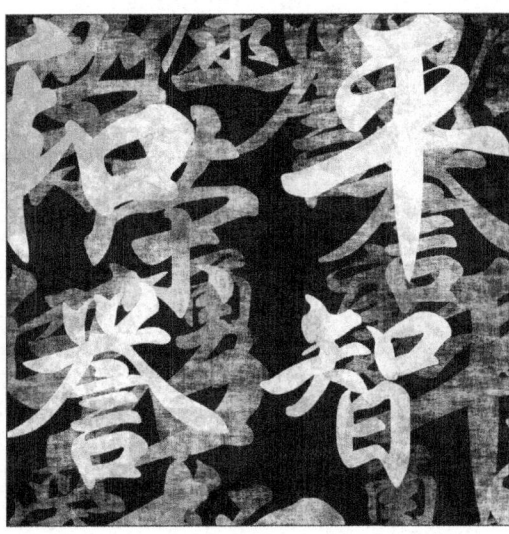

All illustrations courtesy of Dreamstime.com, except where noted.

Introduction

Over ten years ago, as a newly hired faculty member here at the University of California, Berkeley (UCB), I helped coordinate a literacy program combining writing instruction and taekwondo training for fourth graders at an urban, public elementary school in Richmond, California. The program, known as Project Teamwork and co-sponsored by the National Collegiate Athletic Association (NCAA) and the National Writing Project, was a national effort at combining athletic and academic skills development in under-resourced and underperforming educational settings. Like many such efforts, the program was well intentioned and poorly funded. The program likewise had no formal research agenda other than broadly promoting academics through sport in urban American communities. Three other pilot programs were developed as part of Project Teamwork, taking place in Baltimore, Philadelphia, and Mississippi. The Bay Area project was the only pilot program to utilize a martial art as the sport to be combined with academic skill development. One day per week for twelve weeks, twenty-four fourth graders received forty-five minutes of taekwondo training, followed by forty-five minutes of writing instruction.

The program benefited from the voluntary efforts of some well-qualified instructors, as well as several student athletes from UCB, who served as mentors to these young students. The decision to utilize taekwondo as the sport to be paired with academic enrichment rested primarily with Dr. Ken Min, father of UCB's Martial Arts Program (UBMAP).[1] One of the lead authors of the Project Teamwork mission statement and corresponding materials, UCB English Professor Don McQuade, witnessed firsthand the educational and personal benefits of taekwondo when his own son had begun the practice of this martial art under Dr. Min's tutelage. As a result of this relationship and the connection between UBMAP and Project Teamwork, fifth-degree black belt and eight-time national taekwondo heavyweight champion Kim Royce served as these fourth graders' martial arts instructor. Royce had earned both his academic and taekwondo degrees at UCB. Two experienced elementary teachers from Richmond and Oakland, who also were teacher consultants from the Bay Area Writing Project, provided hands-on writing instruction to the students involved in the program. I served as site coordinator and participant observer. I was there to learn how these students learned. As such, I was in charge of documenting the results of the program. This chapter reports these results, reviews the literature, and provides a preliminary analysis of the educational value of taekwondo in one small public school in northern California.

The underlying premise of this project, like many other after-school programs across the United States, was to use athletic participation as an incentive for academic engagement and performance. The vision statement of Project Teamwork attempted to draw this apparent connection between school and sport: "The belief that sport can be used to bind young people's attachment to school and engagement in learning is an article of faith; the United States leads the world in support for scholastic and community sports programs. Scholar athletes across the nation demonstrate that athletics and academics are interrelated arenas for learning where young people can practice, reflect, and advance their skills. The qualities of self-discipline, perseverance, and hard work necessary for excellence in sports are transferable skills available to the young student as much as to the young athlete" (Project Teamwork White Paper, February 25, 1998). So sport would be the hook. Indeed, these fourth graders from Grant Elementary School agreed to stay and write after school in order to kick and punch in novel ways. These mostly African American and Chicano American schoolchildren practiced the discipline of writing while learning the art of taekwondo.

In many instances, these types of extracurricular programs are utilized not merely as an incentive for academic engagement, but as an intervention to combat juvenile delinquency and aggression, manifested in school and street violence. As the mission statement of Project Teamwork attests, the underlying faith in such interventions is that athletic and corporeal training will teach pro-social values such as discipline, respect, and humility. These values, in turn, can be transferred to other facets of life and achievement arenas such as school, where these learned characteristics will help enhance performance. Even more broadly, the physical training associated with sport may increase the participant's self-esteem and sense of control, among other psychological benefits. This commonsense belief that sports build character has been hotly debated in the literature, as has the idea that sports, by their very nature, could decrease delinquency and violence, especially when the activities themselves may appear aggressive and violent to an outside observer. Similarly, the research on the benefit of athletic participation on academic engagement and achievement is likewise mixed. The following seeks to analyze the role of taekwondo training within this literature, focusing in particular on the educational value of the martial art in and of itself, as well as a possible means to other social benefits. Of particular interest is whether the practice of taekwondo might enhance intellectual engagement and academic achievement more effectively than other physical activities, such as more modern, competitive sports. This exploration will perhaps provoke more questions than provide definitive answers. Fourth-grade students from a poor urban school in Richmond, California, help humanize and enrich this research, as these children of color kick and throw punches in the air in a small classroom temporarily turned *dojang* (formal training hall).

A Makeshift Dojang

In white robes cinched tight with white belts around their small frames, a group of ten- and eleven-year-old children kick and shout in unison: *Kiyup! Kiyup!* Their teacher, wearing a far larger white robe with a contrasting black belt instructs: "Now that you're learning taekwondo, you're not learning to fight. You're learning how not to fight."

Taekwondo, often translated as "the way of foot and fist," teaches basic blocking, punching, and kicking techniques, and then combines these elements into more fluid and complex patterns of movement. In its purest form, it is an art of self-defense. The philosophical foundations of taekwondo, however, involve far more than mere physical activity. The *"do"* refers to a moral doctrine, dating back to Confucius, and the active practice of meditation. While the Chinese character *"do"* is a "compound symbol meaning a man's body in the form of walking . . . and another meaning the head, thus inferring that one thinks while walking" (Lee, 2001: 45), the Korean derivation of the word *"do"* is derived from the word meaning "to help" or to educate in finding the way. The dojang, then, is a place for meditation and practice, an educational space for intellectual, physical, even spiritual, training.

At Grant Elementary School, one of the classrooms had become a makeshift dojang for learning the practice of taekwondo on Thursday afternoons. As part of the limited budget of the project, each fourth grader was provided a uniform (*dobok*) with a corresponding belt. In taekwondo, students move through a series of belt levels as their knowledge, skills, and techniques increase. Beginners, such as the fourth graders introduced to this martial art for the first time, wear white belts. Their teacher, Kim Royce, wears a black belt, indicating his advanced level of status and ability. Further levels of expertise are recognized among black belts, from first to tenth *dan* or level rank (Law, 2004). Kim Royce was a black belt, fifth dan.

As evidenced by its inclusion into the Olympic Games, taekwondo can be a competitive martial art. Modern programs emphasize full-contact sparring and self-defense, focused on scoring points and defeating your opponent. Traditional programs focus more heavily on self-control, noncontact sparring, and conflict avoidance, as noted in Royce's initial instruction to the fourth graders. Traditional programs incorporate philosophical teachings and meditation, as well as respect for the instructor (Law, 2004; Nosanchuk, 1981; Nosanchuk and MacNeil, 1989; Trulson, 1986). According to Lee (1989: 58), it is precisely its traditional, philosophical character "which makes Taekwondo an art rather than a mere assortment of physical techniques."[2] The taekwondo training within Project Teamwork emphasized the traditional tenets of the martial art, including self-defense and nonaggression. Kim Royce, who had been both a student and an instructor within the U.C. Berkeley Taekwondo Program, had made this teaching clear from the beginning of the after-school project in Richmond when he told the fourth graders that they were not learning to fight, but to avoid such confrontations. In fact, the ultimate goal of traditional martial arts is seeking never to use the art and eliminate the need for violence altogether (Bäck, 2009).

The emphasis on philosophy and meditation within current forms of taekwondo may well separate it from other modern sports, which focus primarily on physical training and competition. While several authors have celebrated the spiritual and aesthetic possibilities of certain sports (Barthes, 1993; Jackson, 1995; Mitchell, 1997; Pressfield, 2001), traditional training in taekwondo explicitly incorporates these philosophical teachings. It is possible, then, that the philosophical and spiritual aspects of the martial art provide greater opportunity for a more textured learning process, one in which mind and body are trained simultaneously in the dojang. This kinesthetic yet mental training places value in concerted movement, from performing a kick to writing with a pencil, where form is indeed central to performance. The formal patterns (*kata* in Japanese, or *poomse* in Korean), in fact, provide the vehicle for such moral-philosophical training. As Bäck (2009: 230) notes, "martial arts schools hardly ever have philosophy lectures .... Rather, in the spirit of Zen Buddhism, the practitioners are supposed to gain this sort of practical wisdom and spiritual insight via the physical practice itself."

The desired outcome of the activity is likewise critical. Competitive activities or sports that emphasize winning above all else focus primarily on "the attainment of specific psycho-motor outcomes, . . . where [sic] learning and development in both the cognitive and affective domains tend to be secondary, incidental, and not major concerns" (Lombardo, 2000: 2). Where taekwondo develops in character and practice as a modern sport, it may therefore run the risk of straying from the philosophical tenets underlying this traditional martial art. Its potential educational value may also be negatively impacted as a result of this modern development. As such, there may well be a negative relationship between increasing the level of competition in sport and meaningful opportunities for learning, particularly if we value education as promoting open-mindedness or mindfulness. Competition may, in fact, have the opposite effect, closing in on strategy and outcome at the expense of intellectual or spiritual exploration. Of course, this is not solely the case with sport; classrooms and schools in our culture are often structured similarly, teaching to the test, rewarding scores as outcomes rather than fostering learning for learning's sake.

Then again, it may not be the level of competition that poses the problem for learning. It may be an overreliance on training the body at the expense of the mind. In both the classroom and on the playing field, the body functions as a medium for discipline and dominance. That is, the body is a medium of expression, controlled and restricted by the social structure (Douglass, 1978; Mahiri and Van Rheenen, 2010). Educational institutions, while reifying the division of mind and body, likewise train both the physical and pedagogic body. As Watkins (2005: 3-6) demonstrates in her study of the New South Wales education system in Australia, "the school's intention to 'cultivate habits of thoughts and action' could be read as a form of institutional control leading to the production of docile bodies . . . . The pedagogic goal, therefore, was not simply for a child to acquire a body of knowledge but a knowledgeable body: that they had habituated the skills necessary for academic success."

Sport has similarly been used to train the mind and body. Like the official teaching and learning that takes place in schools, sport, too, has an educational function. The education of youth through sport has often been framed as the building of character. Character implies a kind of socio-moral quality, a set of personality attributes befitting a well-adapted, successful social actor. Legendary basketball coach John Wooden's "Pyramid for Success" includes the following character traits: adaptability, alertness, ambition, competitive greatness, condition, confidence, cooperation, enthusiasm, faith, fight, friendship, honesty, industriousness, initiative, integrity, intentness, loyalty, patience, poise, reliability, resourcefulness, self-control, sincerity, skill, and team spirit (Eitzen and Sage, 1986). Feezell (1989: 215) writes, in reference to Wooden's lengthy collection of characteristics, "Not mentioned in this laudable list are wonder, questioning, Socratic ignorance (uncertainty), skepticism, reflectiveness, and critical ability." While not particularly moral or ethical in nature, these latter qualities, if transferred to the classroom, would seem to be valuable in promoting intellectual curiosity and engagement. Advocates of taekwondo claim similar educational and moral values inherent to the traditional martial art. As noted by

Chun (1975: 8; quoted in Law, 2004: 17), "Through strict discipline, taekwondo trains both the mind and body, placing great emphasis on the development of moral character. In other words, control of the mind, self-discipline, kindness and humility must accompany the physical grace." Given the potential psychological benefits of sport, then, these activities have likewise been used as interventions to remedy existing social problems.

After all, educational interventions often presuppose fixing a problem, making some schools and some kids more competitive because they are lagging behind or are "at risk." This was certainly the case with Grant Elementary School in Richmond, California. When we arrived, offering taekwondo training and writing instruction, only 19% of these urban fourth graders scored at the national average of the language section, based on the California's Standardized Testing and Reporting (STAR) scores. Only 11% of these youths scored at the national average in spelling. One question initially, then, was what would be the outcome of this novel, pilot program, other than providing a safe space in a tough neighborhood to practice a martial art and writing? And was anything more needed to justify being there, two large national organizations and a big university coming into this local community, seeking to make a difference in the lives of a couple of dozen youths? Was there something special about taekwondo training, instead of say, basketball, or soccer or swimming, that might add to the desired outcome?

The Case for Taekwondo

In addition to the potential positive academic outcomes, other psychological benefits have been reported as the result of taekwondo training. Some of the reported benefits include enhanced self-esteem and self-confidence (Brown et al., 1995; Duthie, Hope and Barker, 1978; Finkenberg, 1990; Konzak and Bourdeau, 1984; Martin and Pilcher, 1994; Richman and Rehberg, 1986; Trulson, 1986), increased sense of control (Brown et al., 1995; Madden, 1995; Sanson, 1999), and decreased hostility, aggression, and delinquency (Daniels and Thornton, 1992; Lamarre and Nosanchuk, 1999; Nosanchuk, 1981; Skelton, Glynn and Berta, 1991; Trulson, 1986; Twemlow et al., 2008; Zivin et al., 2001).

For example, one of the few studies referred to in the literature supporting sport as a possible treatment for juvenile delinquency uses taekwondo as an intervention. Trulson (1986) identified thirty-four delinquent teenage boys based on the Minnesota Multiphasic Personality Inventory (MMPI) and provided three different protocols three times a week for six months. The first group received training in the traditional Korean martial art of taekwondo, which included philosophical reflection and meditation, in addition to the physical practice of the martial art. The second group received a modern version of taekwondo training, which only included the physical techniques, but without the philosophical teachings of the sport. The third group, which Trulson refers to as the control, participated in a number of other activities, including basketball, football, and jogging.

After six months, the boys were readministered the MMPI. Interestingly, the first group, which had received traditional taekwondo training, showed decreased aggressiveness, lowered anxiety, increased self-esteem, and improved social skills. The scores indicated that these boys were no longer delinquent. Conversely, those boys in the second group who received the modern version of the martial art showed a higher tendency toward delinquency and a marked increase in aggressiveness. The third group of young men showed no difference in delinquency, yet their self-esteem and social skills improved. If one of the research questions under study was whether participation in organized physical activities could have a positive effect on psychological well-being, it seems somewhat odd that this third treatment was described as a control group. While these boys were not receiving taekwondo training in any form, they were participating in sports. The results seem to indicate that this varied sport intervention did indeed have a positive effect on the third group of boys.

These divergent findings demonstrate that sport alone cannot account for providing either social benefits or liabilities. However, the contextual combination of exercising both mind and body within taekwondo training seems to have had the greatest positive impact, at least within this study. As Coakley (2004: 184) notes, "It is unfortunate that Trulson did not include a group receiving the philosophical training without the practice of taekwondo physical skills. Perhaps the integration of philosophical training with physical activity is so effective because the physical activity provides opportunities to 'embody' the philosophy."

Like the first group of boys in Trulson's study, other researchers have found that taekwondo training can decrease aggression in participants, often related to length of training experience (Daniels and Thornton, 1992; Lamarre and Nosanchuk, 1999; Nosanchuk, 1981; Twemlow et al., 2008; Zivin et al., 2001). While some have found an inverse relationship between aggressiveness and level of belt rank

(Skelton, Glynn, and Berta, 1991), Nosanchuk and MacNeil found this relationship to hold only when participants were trained in a traditional martial arts program. These authors found that students attending a modern program became more aggressive as their belt level increased. Thus, the literature draws a clear distinction between modern martial arts, which tend to emphasize competition and aggression, and traditional martial arts instruction, emphasizing the spiritual, psychological, and nonaggressive aspects of training and instruction (Fuller, 1988; Regets, 1990; Trulson, 1986; Twemlow et al., 2008).

Taekwondo and Academic Achievement

While many psychological benefits of traditional taekwondo training have been heralded in the literature, such as enhancing self-esteem, self-confidence, and sense of control, there is very little empirical evidence that such interventions enhance academic engagement and performance. While there is some evidence that martial arts training or interventions in schools may lead to reductions in aggression and delinquency, thereby reducing poor classroom conduct and mandatory principal visits by delinquent children (Lakes and Hoyt, 2004; Smith et al., 1999; Twemlow et al., 2008), it is unclear whether such training translates into higher test scores, grades, and educational achievement. In several studies, however, taekwondo has been shown to help children with Attention-deficit Disorder concentrate more effectively, translating into improved academic engagement and performance (Morand, 2004; Ripley, 2003). While Vockell and Kwak (1990) identify several ways in which skills and knowledge acquired in a taekwondo class can improve academic performance, such as physical safety, mental discipline, and familiarity and comfort in collaborative learning, the authors acknowledge that their assertions are based upon anecdotal evidence.

Such anecdotes or testimonials are common. Perhaps the most cited study of the link between taekwondo training and academic performance, referenced on the websites of numerous private taekwondo academies, is a 1994 article by Martin and Pilcher (http://www.facebook.com/pages/Metairie-LA/Patrick-Lees-Tae KwonDo-Plus/131616210202229; http://www.angelfire. com/sc3/tkdplus/testframe.htm; http://www.tkdtexas.com/stars.php). This study, which looked at 150 nine- to fifteen-year-old students enrolled in taekwondo classes throughout the United States, is not in fact about the effects of martial arts instruction on academic performance, but the effects of such training on preadolescents' and early adolescents' self-esteem. While the results of the study show that students had higher self-esteem after receiving the first cycle of taekwondo training, several websites make the claim that this study found a clear relationship between taekwondo training and increased grades or academic performance. The problem is that this often-cited study does not make such claims. It is not that this relationship does not exist; the literature to date just does not often support a direct correlation between martial arts instruction and improved academic performance. As such, let us return to Richmond, where a group of fourth graders practice their writing after learning the discipline of taekwondo.

Results

In some ways, this after-school program in Richmond offers a cautionary tale against large educational organizations attempting to impact smaller schools and communities with lofty ideals and limited resources. In the 1989 Project Teamwork national document announcing its establishment, the text reads, "Starting with its four pilot sites in Baltimore, Mississippi, Philadelphia and the San Francisco Bay Area, Project Teamwork will expand to a network of twenty sites across the country by 2004 and will support continued expansion to communities with interest and capacity to sustain local programs." Not only did the project not expand to include additional sites; following the pilot year, the initial financial support and commitment to the effort had ended. And yet, while the national effort of Project Teamwork clearly did not meet its targeted goals, the local successes were plentiful. These successes could not necessarily be measured in higher test scores or grades, but they were witnessed in the human spirit of expression.

Writing Taekwondo

When the fourth graders were done with their taekwondo training, they disrobed, folded their uniforms, and bowed as they left their makeshift dojang. The children were now back in their school clothes and entered the real classroom to be instructed in writing, where they were given water and a snack. The teachers wrote some new vocabulary words on the blackboard in front of the classroom. The words were familiar to the fourth graders because they had just been introduced to them during taekwondo training. The new words were spider walk, ax kick, horseback stance, in and out block. Still excited about their martial arts training, the kids would write about taekwondo. The teachers suggested writing a poem about their experience, providing several templates from which the children could choose. They could choose between an ABC poem and a "sandwich poem."

A sandwich poem is a poem that starts with a word, in this case "taekwondo," is followed by several sentences, and then ends with the same word.

Yesenia wrote:

Taekwondo
   Today we did in and out block
   I felt strong and happy
   It's fun to do
   We learn many things
Taekwondo

Angel wrote:

Taekwondo
   The best thing is running
   Building strength
   Kicking, punching
   When I grow up, I want to have a black belt like Mr. Royce
Taekwondo

This theme of respect was reiterated in other poems as well, including an ABC poem written by *Jeanie*:

At taekwondo you
  Bow when you
    Come in the
   Door.
     Every team member
      Follows instruction by the
     Great Master Royce

Fezell added:

Great Master Royce
At taekwondo you
 Bow when entering the Dojang
  Come in quietly
   Give respect to each other
    Jump up and down
     Kick

In a later week, these fourth graders wrote letters to student athletes at UCB, who served as mentors and pen pals to these young martial artists. Students at Grant Elementary School and Berkeley exchanged correspondence, public school students separated by several miles and several years of school. The hope was to inspire these fourth graders to one day attend a university like Berkeley. The fourth graders were asked once again to write about their experiences with taekwondo.

One student, *Angel*, wrote the following letter to his pen pal, Marcus, a varsity football player at UCB:

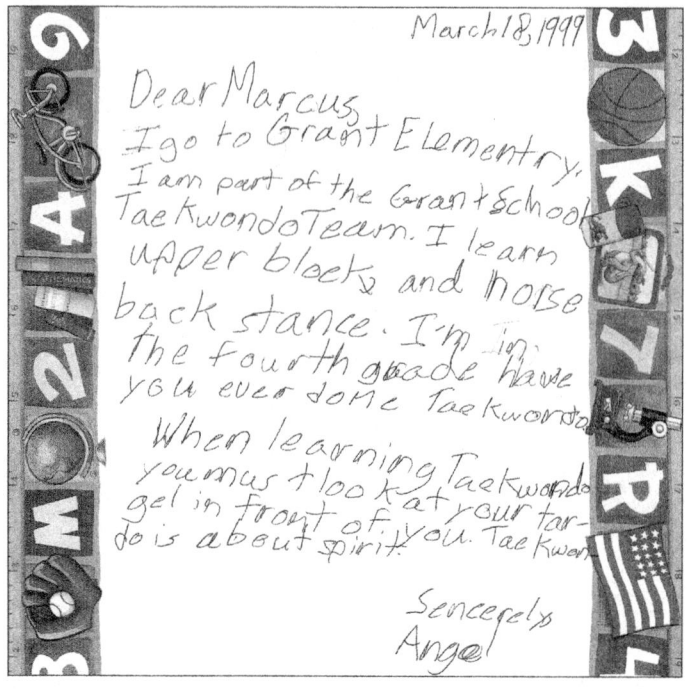

Illustrations courtesy of D. Van Rheenen.

The letter reads (with misspellings left intact):

March 18, 1999

Dear Marcus,
I go to Grant Elementary.
I am part of the Grant School
Taekwondo Team. I learn
upper blocks and horse
back stance. I'm in
the fourth grade Have
you ever done Taekwondo.
When learning Taekwondo
you must look at your tar-
gel in front of you. Taekwondo is about spirit.

Sencerely,
Angel

The written words of these fourth graders captured a sense of their engagement in learning taekwondo, expressing how they felt strong and happy. The youths articulated respect for the spirit of the activity, respect for the space where the learning and training took place, and respect for their teacher. The fourth graders wrote about their sense of pride in being part of the Grant Elementary School Taekwondo team. Of note was that these urban youths wrote about something they liked to do. And they wrote once the school bell marking the end of formal instruction had sounded.

Once the pilot monies dried up, the writing teachers affiliated with the National Writing Project left. The student athlete mentors lost contact with the elementary school students, no longer exchanging letters with the Richmond youths. I returned to the comfort of my office as a faculty member at UCB, moving on to new projects. The Grant School Taekwondo Team persevered, however. By an act of tremendous good fortune, the taekwondo instructor, Master Kim Royce, became a fourth-grade teacher at Grant. He met his future wife at Grant. They had a son, now five years old, whose middle name is Grant, in honor of the school where his father and mother taught other kids. Under his leadership and with the support of the principal at the time (there have been four different principals at Grant since he began teaching fourth grade there), he helped turn a bungalow in the middle of the playground into a semipermanent dojang. The Grant School Taekwondo Team continued to flourish, competing at the UC Open Championships for the past ten years. Royce estimates that he has now coached several hundred elementary schoolchildren as part of the Grant school team.

Despite the many positive results following this after-school literacy program, it may appear that there is limited empirical evidence demonstrating a positive effect of taekwondo participation on academic achievement. For example, if we analyze California's standardized test scores for elementary schoolchildren at Grant Elementary over the past decade, we do not find appreciable improvements. Granted, the writing instruction in the after-school program only lasted one year, but we might expect that taekwondo participation alone would suffice to make a difference in academic performance. Does this mean that introduction to the martial art was of little to no benefit to these elementary schoolchildren?

Because pre- and post-tests of psychological well-being were not assessed as a part of this study, it is difficult to identify the potential benefits of participation in this martial arts program. And because we have not tracked the participants longitudinally, we cannot say at this point whether these youths benefited in a meaningful way regarding their self-esteem, confidence, academic performance, and educational aspirations. The discussion does suggest that future research is warranted, not only on the taekwondo participants at Grant Elementary School, but also on taekwondo participants throughout the United States and elsewhere.

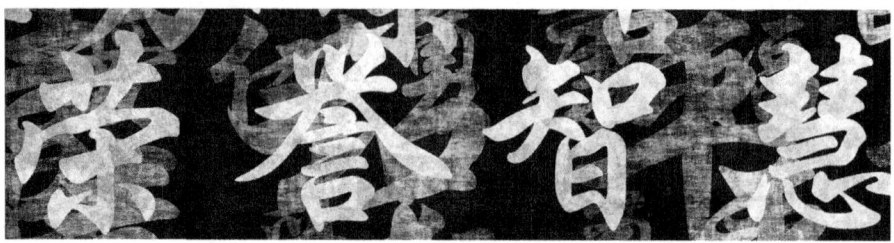

Implications and Future Directions for Research

If we take these children at their word, their written word that is, the fourth graders at Grant Elementary School learned a lot in just twelve weeks. In addition to learning a horseback stance, they learned to respect others and ultimately themselves. They discovered that learning could be fun, even if it required a lot of hard work. Because the Grant Taekwondo School Team continued after the initial pilot year, many of these fourth graders continued to practice this martial art. To expect that this novel program and introduction to taekwondo would alter the disparities in even one of California's public schools would be naïve. The challenges are formidable. But these fourth graders, ages ten and eleven at the time of Project Teamwork, are now in their early twenties. One area of potential research, then, is to rediscover these young men and women and interview them about how and in what ways taekwondo changed their perspectives toward learning and school, toward the world in which they live. As had been hoped for at the time of the project, it would be interesting to determine how many of these youths went on to graduate from high school. Similarly, it would be worth investigating just how many of these fourth graders from 1999 are now completing college or have earned a baccalaureate degree. If so, it would be worth determining if lessons learned in the dojang influenced their attitude and behaviors toward school and education.

Given the limited number of studies that directly address the relationship of taekwondo and school success, this is an area of future research. That self-esteem and self-reliance improve as a result of practicing this martial art, it is quite likely that these qualities will in turn positively affect academic competence and confidence. The studies simply need to be designed. If we study students who choose to participate in taekwondo independently, rather than as an intervention, we must proceed with caution. The individuals who elect to participate in martial arts in the first place may possess qualities or characteristics conducive to academic achievement. If, for example, we were to look at the general student body at any particular institution that offers martial arts training, comparing martial artists with nonparticipants, we would need to control for like factors, including academic profile (GPA and test scores), family background, income, and parents' education. But where these demographic and cognitive factors are roughly the same, we can then analyze the possible effect that martial art participation has on academic performance, major selection, time to degree, ultimate career choice, and so on. There may well be differences among martial artists as well, differences by level of proficiency or belt, and differences by type of the martial art itself. These types of studies would allow us also to test a proposition introduced in this chapter: whether martial arts in general, and taekwondo in particular, have different effects regarding academic performance than other sports might have. This would suggest a possible study at colleges or universities, contrasting martial artists with other club sports participants or varsity student athletes. Again, the same cautions and caveats hold as to controlling for other factors influencing differences in tested outcomes.

To be sure, the effects of taekwondo training on elementary, middle-school, and high-school students is also worthy of study. As this chapter has attempted to demonstrate, Grant Elementary School benefited from having a fourth-grade teacher who happened to be a black belt and a phenomenal teacher, both in the classroom and in the dojang. More schools would benefit from including taekwondo in their educational curriculum. I caution to say that taekwondo training should be included as part of schools' physical education curriculum, not only because physical educational programs across the state and country have been decimated in recent years but, perhaps more important, because taekwondo is far more than simply physical education. At least as a traditional practice, taekwondo is a training of mind and body, an exploration of consciousness. This consciousness recognizes embodiment and works to deconstruct the classical Cartesian division of mind and body.

Clearly there is a need to practice the teaching of a more balanced approach to mind and body work. This approach suggests recognizing the mental discourse of all sport, such as seen in taekwondo, as well as the physical nature of learning. Understanding and valuing a kinesthetic style of learning could promote a similar somatic style of teaching in the classroom. Here coaches and teachers of all disciplines have much to learn from the traditional tenets of taekwondo. For example, we might begin to highlight the roles of the student body assisting, rather than competing against, one another. Such a mindset could help to create a more positive and collaborative learning environment in both school and sport. A shift toward a safer, more respectful space for learning requires that we not position youths in ways that limit their potential, put them at risk, and stifle opportunities for success. As a nation, we need to change the way we see the relationship of sport and school. We need to include rather than exclude, to redefine measures of success, and to offer more, rather than fewer, opportunities for personal growth. It appears to me that the practice of taekwondo has known for a very long time how to teach these values to children and adults alike.

[1] As noted on their website (http://www.ucmap.org/about.php), "since its inception in 1969, the Martial Arts Program of the University of California's Berkeley campus has had a twofold mission. In addition to providing successful, quality technical instruction in all martial arts/sports, the UC Martial Arts Program also endeavors to maximize the academic resources of the university to develop martial arts/sports through research into their philosophical, spiritual and scientific implications." Project Teamwork, and this chapter about the after-school project, are consistent with the mission of UBMAP.

[2] For an interesting discussion of the moral distinctions between the practice of traditional martial arts and participation in modern sports, see Bäck (2009: 217-237).

REFERENCES

Bäck, A. (2009). The way to virtue in sport. *Journal of the Philosophy of Sport*, 36, 217-237.

Barthes, R. (1993). *Mythologies*. London: Vintage.

Beaumont Taekwondo and Jiu-Jitsu Academy website. Retrieved August 18, 2010 from http://www.tkdtexas.com/stars.php.

Brown, D., Wang, Y., Ward, A., Ebbeling, C., Fortlage, L., Puleo, E., Benson, H. and Rippe, J. (1995). Chronic psychological effects of exercise and exercise plus cognitive strategies. *Medicine and Science in Sports and Exercise*, 27(5), 765-775.

Charles Newton's Taekwondo Plus website. Retrieved August, 17, 2010 from http://www.angelfire.com/sc3/tkdplus/testframe.htm.

Coakley, J. (2004). *Sports in society: Issues and controversies*. Boston: McGraw-Hill.

Daniels, K. and Thornton, E. (1992). Length of training, hostility and the martial arts: A comparison with other sporting groups. *British Journal of Sports Medicine*, 26, 118-120.

Douglas, M. (1978). *Natural symbols*. New York: Praeger.

Duthie, R., Hope, L. and Barker, D. (1978). Selected personality traits of martial artists as measured by the adjective checklist. *Journal of Perceptual and Motor Skills*, 47, 71-76.

Eitzen, D. and Sage, G. (Eds.). *Sociology of Northern American*, 3rd Edition. Dubuque, Iowa: Wm. C. Brown Publishers.

Feezell, R. (1989, Fall). Sport, character, and virtue. *Philosophy Today*, 33, 204-220.

Finkenberg, M. (1990). Effect of participation in taekwondo on college women's self-concept. *Journal of Perceptual and Motor Skills*, 71, 891-894.

Fuller, J. (1988). Martial arts and psychological health. *British Journal of Medical Psychology*, 61(4), 317-328.

Jackson, P. (1995). *Sacred hoops: Spiritual lessons of a hardwood warrior*. New York: Hyperion.

Konzak, B. and Bourdeau, F. (1984). Martial arts training and mental health: An exercise in self-help. *Canada's Mental Health*, 32(4), 2-8.

Lakes, K. and Hoyt, W. (2004) Promoting self-regulation through school-based martial arts training. *Applied Developmental Psychology*, 25(3), 283-302.

Lamarre, B. and Nosanchuk, T. (1999). Judo—The gentle way: A replication of studies on martial arts and aggression. *Journal of Perceptual and Motor Skills*, 88, 992-996.

LAW, D. (2004). A choice theory perspective on children's taekwondo. *International Journal of Reality Therapy, 24*, 13-18.

LEE, K. (2001). *Taekwondo: Philosophy and culture*. Elizabeth, NJ: Hollym.

LEE, T. (1989). *Mastering taekwondo*. Ottawa, Ontario, Canada: Tae Eun Lee.

LOMBARDO, B. (2000). Coaching in the 21st century: Issues, concerns and solutions. *Sosol: Sociology of Sport Online*, 1-3.

MADDEN, M. (1995). Perceived vulnerability and control of martial arts and physical fitness students. *Journal of Perceptual and Motor Skills, 80*(3), 899–910.

MAHIRI, J. AND D. VAN RHEENEN (2010). *Out of bounds: When scholarship athletes become academic scholars*. Studies in the Postmodern Theory of Education, Vol. 363. New York: Peter Lang.

MARTIN, W. AND PILCHER, J. (Fall 1994). The effects of martial arts instruction on preadolescents' and early adolescents' self-esteem. *Journal of Research in Education, 4*(1), 1-3.

MITCHELL, R. (1997). *The Tao of sports*. Berkeley: Frog, Ltd.

MORAND, M. (2004). The effects of mixed martial arts on behavior of male children with attention deficit hyperactivity disorder. Unpublished dissertation. Hofstra University, Hampstead, N.Y.

NOSANCHUK, T. (1981). The way of the warrior: The effects of traditional martial arts training on aggressiveness. *Human Relations, 34*(6), 435-444.

NOSANCHUK, T., AND MACNEIL, C. (1989). Examination of the effects of traditional and modern martial arts training on aggressiveness. *Aggressive Behavior, 15*, 153-159.

PATRICK LEE'S TAEKWONDO PLUS website. Retrieved August 17, 2010 from http://www.facebook.com/pages/Metairie-LA/Patrick-Lees-TaeKwonDo-Plus/131616210202229

PRESSFIELD, S. (2001). *The legend of Bagger Vance: A novel of golf and the game of life*. London: Bantam Books.

REGETS, C. (1990). The relationship between self-actualization and levels of involvement in aikido. ProQuest Dissertation Abstracts. AAC 9027839.

RICHMAN, C. AND REHBERG, H. (1986). The development of self-esteem through the martial arts. *International Journal of Sport Psychology, 17*(3), 234-239.

RIPLEY, A. (2003). An awesome alternative to drugs: Martial arts practice as treatment for children with AD/HD. Retrieved 18th August 2010 from http://www.capella.edu/portal/alumni/scontent/ProfOpp/

SANSONE, M. (1999). Taekwondo achievement and locus of control. M.A. Thesis, Rowan University.

SKELTON, D., GLYNN, M. AND BERTA, S. (1991). Aggressive behavior as a function of taekwondo ranking. *Perceptual and Motor Skills, 72*(1), 179-182.

SMITH, J., TWEMLOW, S., AND HOOVER, D. (1999). Bullies, victims and bystanders: A method of in-school intervention and possible parental contributions. *Child Psychiatry and Human Development, 30*(1), 29-37.

TRULSON, M. (1986). Martial arts training: A novel "cure" for juvenile delinquency. *Human Relations, 39*(12), 1131-1140.

TWEMLOW, S., BIGGS, B., NELSON, T., VERNBER, E., FONAGY, P. AND TWEMLOW, S. (2008). Effects of participation in a martial arts–based antibullying program in elementary schools. *Psychology in the Schools, 45*(10), 947-959.

TWEMLOW, S. AND SACCO, F. (1998). The application of traditional martial arts practice and theory to the treatment of violent adolescents. *Adolescence, 33*(131), 505-518.

UNIVERSITY OF CALIFORNIA, BERKELEY MARTIAL ARTS PROGRAM website. Retrieved October 14, 2010 from http://www.ucmap.or/about.php

VOCKELL, E. AND KWAK, H. (1990). Martial arts in the classroom. *The Clearing House, 64*(1), 61-63.

WATKINS, M. (June, 2005). The erasure of habit: Tracing the pedagogic body. *Discourse: Studies in the Cultural Politics of Education, 26*(2), 167-181.

ZIVIN, G., HASSAN, N., DEPAULA, G., MONTI, D., HARLAN, C., HOSSAIN, K. AND PATTERSON, K. (2001). An effective approach to violence prevention: Traditional martial arts in middle school. *Adolescence, 36*(143), 443-459.

chapter 8

Teaching Aikido to Children with Autism Spectrum Disorders

by Josh Paul, M.A.

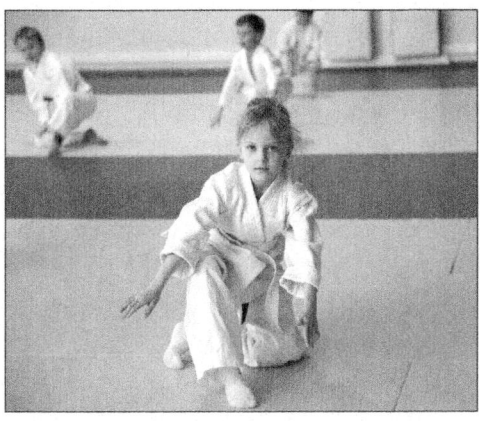

Photograph courtesy of Dreamstime.com

Introduction

Martial arts are paths of physical, intellectual, spiritual, and social growth. Among children, adolescents, and college students, martial arts training is associated with reductions in inappropriate social behaviors, violence, and aggression (Daniels and Thorton, 1992; Lamarre and Nosancuk, 1999; Woodward, 2009; Zivin et al., 2001), as well as increased prosocial behaviors, improved classroom conduct, and improved sleep quality, mood, and mental health (Caldwell, Harrison, Adams, and Triplett, 2009; Lakes and Hoyt, 2004; Wang, 2008; Woodward, 2009). Although the research is limited, there is evidence that martial arts also improve confidence, self-esteem, and quality of life among children with intellectual and physical disabilities (Conant, Morgan, Muzykewicz, Clark, and Thiele, 2008; Gleser et al., 1992; Wall, 2005; Woodward, 2009; Wright, White, and Gaebler-Spira, 2004).

Autism spectrum disorders (ASD) are the second–most-common developmental disability in the United States, affecting more children than childhood cancers, juvenile diabetes, and pediatric AIDS combined, and the prevalence of ASD is increasing 10–17% annually (Autism Speaks, 2011a). As the prevalence of ASD increases, martial arts instructors will be increasingly faced with the question of whether to enroll children with ASD in their dojo and how to best teach this population. Aikido, and martial arts in general, have the potential to fill many of the psychosocial needs of this special population by providing a recreational activity that fosters intellectual, physical, and social growth, as well as much-needed "normal" childhood experiences.

Since 2007 I have taught short-term aikido courses to children with medium- and high-functioning ASD and other developmental disabilities enrolled in New York City public schools. Through a process of trial and error, I developed a cumulative curriculum of selected aikido exercises that emphasize focus, body awareness, and awareness of others. This chapter provides a background on ASD, and, based my experiences, discusses general considerations and curriculum for teaching children with ASD. Although the curriculum presented is specifically aikido based, the exercises could be adapted to any martial arts environment.

Autism Spectrum Disorders: Facts and Figures

In the broadest sense, ASD are a group of developmental disorders characterized by difficulties in communication and social interaction (Brasic, 2011). Autism is considered a "spectrum" disorder because of the extraordinary variability in the type and severity of symptoms and behaviors (Table 1).

According to a 2009 study from the Centers for Disease Control and Prevention (CDC), which reviewed medical records for eight-year-olds in eleven U.S. cities, 1 out of every 110 children, or nearly 1% of all children, in the United States is on the autistic spectrum (CDC, 2009). The study also found that the prevalence of ASD increased 57% between 2002 and 2006. This increase was partly attributed to changes and improvements in screening systems, diagnostic methods, and broadened definitions, but part of the increase represented real growth in the number of children with ASD.

A more recent study reported an even higher prevalence (Kim et al., 2011). This study screened all children ages seven to twelve years old (approximately 55,000) in a single community in South Korea rather than reviewing medical records. Using this methodology, the investigators found a prevalence of 2.64%, equivalent to approximately 1 in 38 children. The findings suggest that the prevalence in the United States might be higher than currently thought if calculated using a similar method.

ASD occur in both genders, and all racial, ethnic, and socioeconomic groups, but are four to five times more common in boys than girls (CDC, 2009; CDC, 2011). An estimated 1 in 70 boys and 1 in 310 girls are affected (CDC, 2009). ASD are also frequently associated with intellectual disability: 41% of children with ASD have an IQ of 70 or less (a normal IQ is considered between 90 and 109) (CDC, 2011).

Autism Spectrum Disorders: Categories, Diagnosis, and Treatment

There are three broad categories of ASD: autistic disorder (classic autism), Asperger syndrome, and pervasive developmental disorder (CDC, 2011). Autistic disorder is characterized by profound difficulties with language, communication, and social interactions. Children and adults with autistic disorder often exhibit unusual behaviors and interests, and it is frequently accompanied by intellectual disabilities and other conditions, such as seizures, Down syndrome, and mental health issues.

Like autistic disorder, Asperger syndrome is characterized by difficulties with social interaction and communication, but not the speech problems or intellectual disabilities typical of autistic disorder (CDC, 2011). Children and adults with Asperger syndrome are usually socially awkward with tendencies to engage in one-sided conversations and exhibit unusual nonverbal communication. They may appear to lack empathy or connection with others, and may have obsessive, narrow interests, among other qualities (Table 2) (Mayo Clinic, 2010; CDC, 2011).

The third category—pervasive development disorders (PDD)—is a nonspecific description of children and adults with some, but not all, of the characteristics of autistic disorder or Asperger syndrome. The symptoms, severity, and intellectual disabilities among those with PDD are variable, but most have social difficulties and unexpected responses to noises, lights, and other sensory information (NINDS, 2011).

ASD are diagnosed by observation and evaluation. There are no blood tests or imaging studies. The disorders are detectable very early—symptoms appear within the first one to two years of life—and a trained physician can reliably diagnose ASD by age two (CDC, 2011). Treatment of ASD consists of multiple types of behavioral therapies designed to improve communication and social skills and intellectual abilities (Autism Speaks, 2011b). Different diets (e.g., gluten-free diets) have been associated with reductions in symptom severity, at least temporarily, as has regular exercise. Medications can be used to treat specific symptoms or associated conditions (e.g., depression and anxiety) (Autism Speaks, 2011b). Interventions started early in life produce the best results.

ASD and Aikido

Like all children, those with ASD and other developmental disabilities experience emotional and psychiatric problems. Depression, anxiety, low self-esteem, and feelings of isolation and unmet needs for intimacy are common (Lundström et al., 2011; Mukaddes, Herüner, and Tanidir, 2010; Müller, Schuler, and Yates, 2008; Sebastian, Blakemore, and Charman, 2009; Twyman et al., 2010; Vickerstaff, Heriot, Wong, Lopes, and Dossetor, 2007). Children with ASD and other disabilities are more likely to be bullied, victimized, and ostracized than other children (Twyman et al., 2010), which can precipitate or exacerbate already existing self-esteem and emotional issues. What is sometimes misunderstood is that although children with ASD may not demonstrate or express a need for social belonging or connection, they do in fact have such needs, and many children with ASD aspire to be productive members of a community and develop social skills and friendships (Müller, Schuler, and Yates, 2008).

Compounding such social challenges are physical challenges: children with ASD and other disabilities are two to three times more likely to be obese than the general population, and more likely to suffer from illnesses and emotions secondary to obesity such as high blood pressure, high cholesterol, depression, fatigue, and low self-esteem (Rimmer, et al, 2010). Also, unlike their counterparts without special needs, children with ASD spend an extraordinary amount of time in therapy.

Within this psychosocial context, there is a clear and pressing need for recreational activities like martial arts that promote community and social interaction, as well as hold the potential to improve physical and psychological health. Aikido, as a physical practice, develops balance, coordination, body awareness, focus, and sensitivity to others. As a path of personal development, it encourages nonverbal and verbal connection and communication, collective learning, community involvement, and self-awareness. And, like all martial arts, aikido has the potential to improve self-esteem and overall mental health.

Considerations for Teachers

Children with ASD are diverse, with unique and sometimes unexpected behaviors warranting some special considerations. The most consistent characteristic of children with ASD is that they do not (cannot) always follow or respond to verbal instructions. At times, it may look and feel as if a student is ignoring you or deliberately looking past you, but this is emblematic of ASD. Other times the same student may seem completely present (like everybody, children with ASD have good and bad days). Special efforts such as physical touch, repeating a student's name, standing next to the student, and other strategies may be needed to elicit responses and focus.

As might be expected, children with ASD have difficulty understanding and engaging in partner practice, which is the core of aikido practice. Although part of a typical aikido class includes group stretching and exercises, most of the practice is done with a partner, with each person alternating between *uke* and *nage* (attacker and defender, respectively). There is very little individual kata practice in aikido. Among children with a disorder specifically characterized by difficulties in communication and relating to others, establishing partner practice is difficult, and may require more diligence than with other students. The instructor cannot simply say, "Get a partner" and expect something to happen. However, the physical, verbal, and nonverbal communication that occurs during practice is part of the uniqueness of the experience.

Teaching and maintaining partner practice ultimately requires more individualized attention, and classes may require a higher teacher-to-student ratio than other classes. Teenaged teaching assistants are an option, as are parents, guardians, and siblings. Additional supervisors do not have to be practitioners of the art being taught, as long as they understand how to maintain class structure. Likewise, when enrolling new students, keep the parents/guardians/therapists—whoever brings the student to class—in the dojo until you feel comfortable and confident.

Talking with parents, guardians, siblings, therapists, and teachers (if possible) is important too, as children with ASD and other disabilities may have unique health risks that could endanger their safety in a martial arts class. For example, up to 30% of people with Down syndrome have a structural deformity at the base of the skull known as atlantoaxial instability, which increases the risk of neck and spinal cord injuries (Alvarez, 2010). Other behaviors to be aware of include unexpected reactions to lights, noises, colors, and shapes, issues with physical contact, and behavioral issues/aggression. Ask questions about individual needs, risks, and behaviors more than once and on an ongoing basis. Children and adults with ASD are not static; symptoms and symptom severity change over time. If you have any doubts, concerns, or questions, do your own research and find your own answers. Table 3 lists some reliable resources.

What to Teach?

What to teach children with ASD? The short answer: aikido (or another martial art), but in small, sequential steps, using exercises that cater to the needs of the students. Over the course of multiple short-term programs (five to twelve weeks), I tried many standard aikido exercises—*aiki taiso* (ki exercise), *tai sabaki toshu* (basic body movements against various attacks), strikes (*shomenuchi, munetsuki, yokomenuchi*), *kokyudosa, shikko* walking, *ukemi*, etc. I eventually found a core group that students were able to successfully perform after a few classes. These were accepted as recognizable martial techniques (students responded better to movements they had seen in movies or computer games), and they were fun.

Aiki taiso exercises, also called ki exercises, are a series of exercises developed by Tohei Koichi (1920–2011) designed to improve body awareness, posture, breath control, focus, balance, and coordination. They also serve as the building blocks of techniques. There are more than a dozen ki exercises, but, at least at the beginning of a program, I focus on six of them (Figures 1–6):

1) unbendable arm (*orenaite*)
2) rowing (*funakogi*)
3) blocking (*shomenuchi ikkyo*)
4) pivoting (*zengo*)
5) turning (*tenkan*)
6) rolling backward and forward (*koho tento*)

* Note: For complete descriptions of all the ki exercises, see Shifflett, 2000.

Figure 1: Unbendable Arm (*orenaite*).
Maintaining a relaxed but unbendable arm is important for blocking and deflecting, rolling, and controlling an attacker. To test orenaite, have a student stand in a front stance and press down on the elbow and up on the wrist simultaneously. Students wiggle their fingers to demonstrate relaxation.

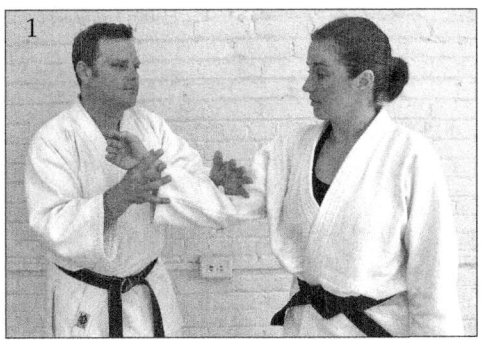

Figure 2: Rowing Exercise (*funakogi undo*).
This is a four-step exercise. From a front stance: hips rock forward and arms extend (2a); hips rock backward and arms retract (2b). The arms should make a small figure eight, as if rowing a boat. Rowing exercise performed with a partner (2c). Hands should just touch when students row forward. To perform dynamically, have students face each other and perform the exercise with one student stepping forward and the other backward.

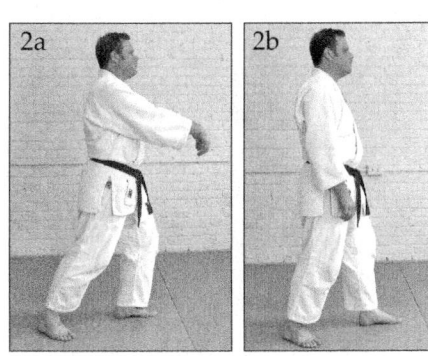

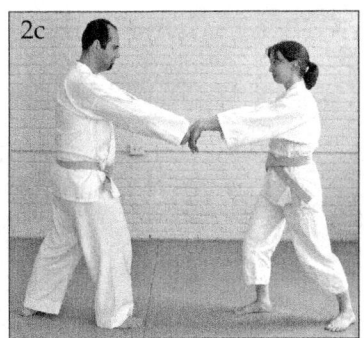

Figure 3: Blocking–Deflecting Exercise (*shomenuchi ikkyo undo*).
This is a four-step exercise. From a front stance: hips rock forward; unbendable arms rise from shoulders (3a), unbendable arms drop, and hips rock back to a neutral front stance. Blocking–deflecting exercise performed with a partner (3b). Partners work in unison. Fingertips should just touch when arms are in the raised position. To perform dynamically, have students face each other and perform the exercise with one student stepping forward and the other backward.

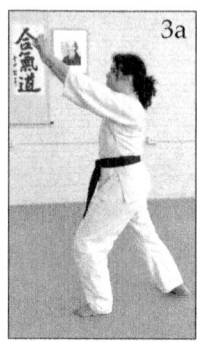 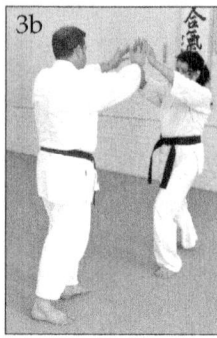

Figure 4: Pivoting Exercise (*zengo undo*).
This exercise is the blocking–deflecting exercise, but performed in two directions. There is a 180° pivot between each blocking movement. When performed with a partner, the fingertips should just touch. In this picture, *zengo undo* is practiced with multiple people in a circle. This requires students to maintain spacing in two directions.

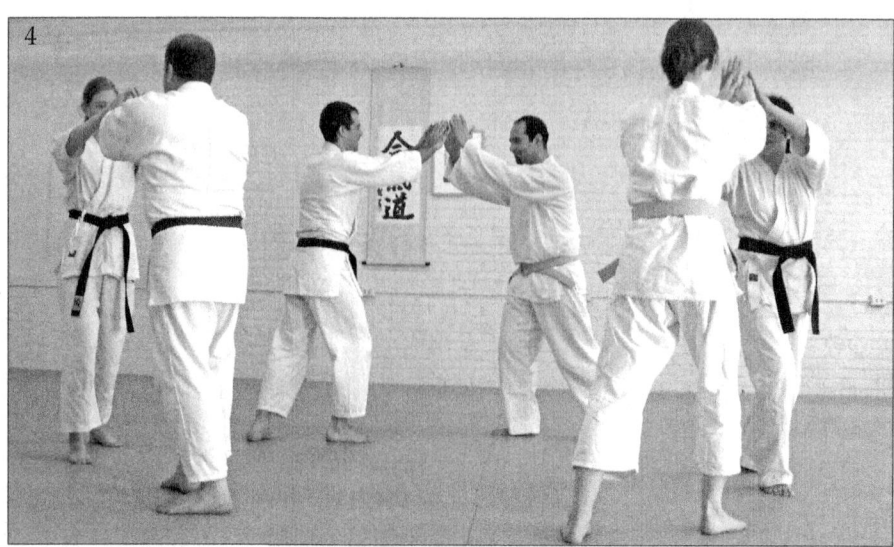

Figure 5: Turning Exercise (*tenkan undo*).
This is a two-step turning exercise. From a front stance, the student turns 180° on the front foot (5a–c). The movement is repeated, continuing in the same direction, to return to the start position.

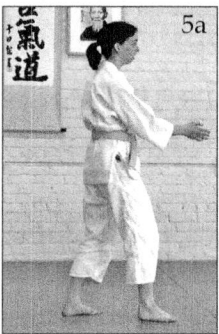
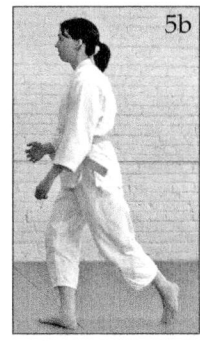
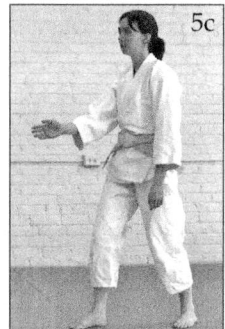

Figure 6a-c: Rolling Exercise (*koho tento undo*)
From a position kneeling on one knee, students roll back and return to the seat position. The same can be performed from kneeling and standing positions. When performed from standing, students kneel, roll back, kneel, and return to a front stance. Make sure hands are kept in front, and not used to stop the roll.

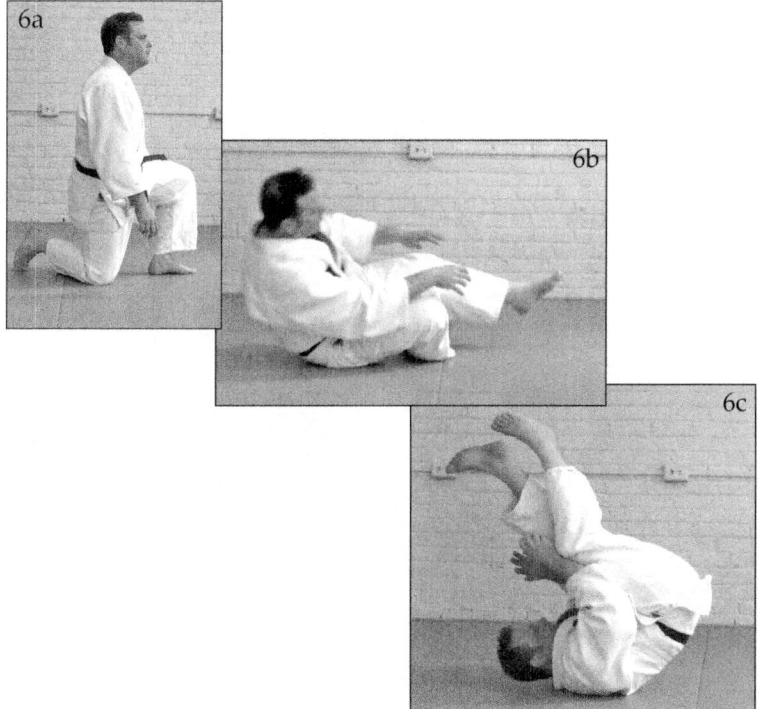

Figure 7a: Forward Roll (*koho tento*).
Figure 7b: Backward Roll (*koho tento kaiten*).

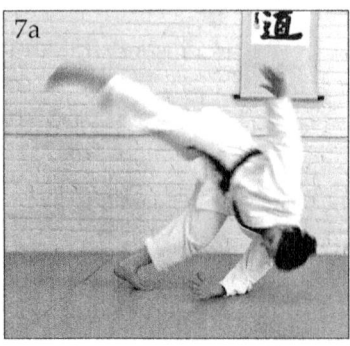
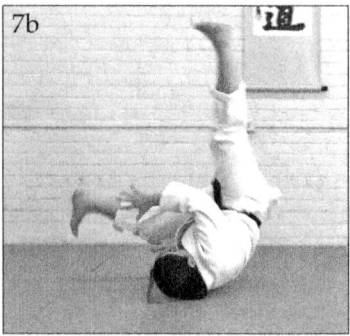

Figure 8: Knee Walking (*shikko*).
This exercise emphasizes movement from the hips, is fun, and usually easily learned by children. Have students start by sitting in *seiza*, lifting one foot and placing it squarely on the floor (8a), and pushing the knee all the way down while simultaneously rotating on the opposite knee (8b). Rather than reach out with the foot and leg, the rotation pushes the leg out from the hip.

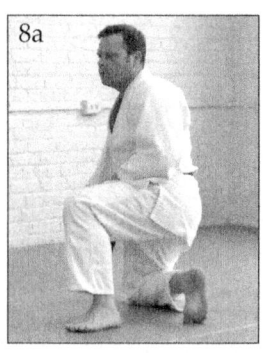
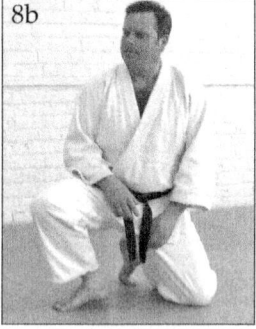

Figure 9: Escaping from Wrist Grabs.

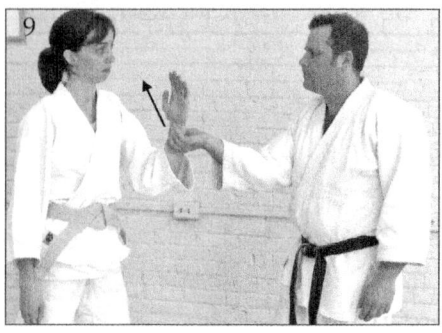

Figure 10: Breathing Exercise (*kokyudosa*).
There are many variations to this exercise. In the one shown, partners sit on their leg (*seiza*), their knees barely touching, with the attacker holding the other's wrists (10a). The defender separates her arms and extends up, toward the attacker's head, lifting her center. She then turns slightly to throw the attacker (10b).

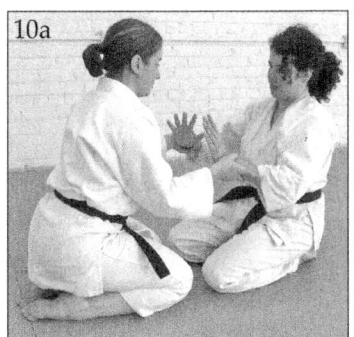
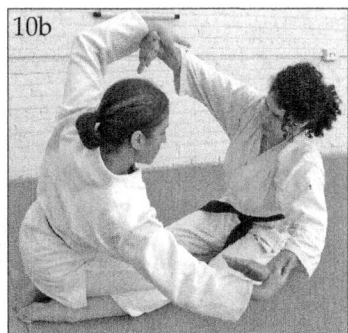

Ki exercises are particularly useful when teaching children with ASD. In addition to the primary intent of developing body awareness, coordination, etc., ki exercises can be performed solo and with a partner, and statically and dynamically (that is, standing still and with motion). They provide a vehicle for safely introducing partner practice while improving balance and coordination, and by checking balance during the practice (ki testing) the exercises provide feedback about a student's body awareness and coordination. Unlike tai sabaki toshu exercises, there is no uke or nage when performing partnered ki exercises—each person does the same thing—making the partner aspect more comprehensible. Other well-received individual practices are *ukemi* (backward and forwards roll) and *shikko* (knee) walking (Figures 7-8).

I continue partner practice and introduce uke/nage roles with escaping from grips (wrist and maybe lapel holds) and kokyudosa (Figures 9 and 10). In this latter exercise, partners sit on their legs (*seiza*) with knees barely touching. Uke holds nage's wrists, and nage tries to unbalance uke by stretching uke beyond her balance point (this should not be a wrestling match). The practice teaches each participant about his or her balance and coordination. Kokyudosa can then be performed standing as the students' first throwing technique (*kokyunage*), and as skills are acquired and improved, more can be introduced.

This curriculum is not a therapeutic intervention; however, there is ongoing research into using an aikido curriculum as a therapeutic option (Kramer, 2011). Although I have had repeated success with this format, there is no guarantee that this approach will work with all students, in all environments, and for all instructors. It can and should be adapted to individual circumstances and students.

Instructor Expectations and Conclusions

Children with ASD are all different and change over time. They should not be expected to conform to any specified set of expectations or requirements. As instructors, it is important that our expectations be flexible and our teaching style responsive and observant. Some extra patience will be required when teaching this unique population, and given the diversity among children with ASD, some trial and error should be expected. As the prevalence of ASD increases, recreational activities like aikido and other martial arts that foster physical, social, and emotional health will be increasingly important.

Table 1: Common Autistic Behaviors

- Not responding to name by 12 months
- Not pointing at objects to show interest by 14 months
- Not playing "pretend" games by 18 months
- Avoiding eye contact and wanting to be alone
- Having trouble understanding other people's feelings or talking about their own feelings
- Delayed speech and language skills
- Repeating words or phrases over and over (echolalia)
- Giving unrelated answers to questions
- Getting upset by minor changes
- Obsessive interests
- Flapping hands, rocking bodies, spinning in circles
- Unusual reactions to sounds, smells, tastes, or how things look or feel

SOURCE: Centers for Disease Control and Prevention.
Facts about Autism Spectrum Disorders. Retrieved May 25, 2011, from http://www.cdc.gov/ncbddd/autism/facts.html.

Table 2: Common Behaviors Among Children & Adults with Asperger Syndrome
• Trouble understanding other people's feelings and talking about their own • Difficulty understanding body language • Avoiding eye contact • Wanting to be alone; or wanting to interact, but not knowing how • Narrow, sometimes obsessive, interests • Talking only about themselves and their interests • Speaking in unusual ways or with an odd tone of voice. • Difficulty making friends. • Appearing nervous in large social groups. • Clumsy or awkward • Rituals that they refuse to change, such as a very rigid bedtime routine • Developing odd or repetitive movements • Unusual sensory reactions. SOURCE: Centers for Disease Control and Prevention. Asperger Syndrome Fact Sheet. Retrieved May 25, 2011, from ww.cdc.gov/ncbddd/actearly/pdf/parents_pdfs/Asperger_Syndrome.pdf.

Table 3: Additional resources for learning about ASD	
Autism Collaboration	www.autism.org
Autism Research Institute	www.autism.com
Autism Science Foundation	www.autismsciencefoundation.org
Autism Society of America	www.autism-society.org
Autism Speaks	www.autismspeaks.org
Centers for Disease Control & Prevention	cdc.gov/ncbddd/autism/index.html
Medscape	www.medscape.com/resource/autism
National Autism Association	www.nationalautismassociation.org
National Inst. of Neurological Disorders & Stroke	www.ninds.nih.gov
U.S. Autism and Asperger Association	www.usautism.org
WebMD	www.webmd.com/brain/autism/default.htm

REFERENCES

Alvarez, A. (2010). Atlantoaxial instability in Down syndrome. Retrieved May 18, 2011, from http://emedicine.medscape.com/article/1180 354-overview.

Autism Speaks (2011a). What is autism? Retrieved May 18, 2011, from http://www.autismspeaks.org/whatisit/index.php.

Autism Speaks (2011b). Treating autism. Retrieved May 18, 2011, from http://www.autismspeaks.org/treatment/index.php.

Brasic, J. (2011). Autism. Retrieved May 17, 2011, from http://emedicine.medscape.com/article/912781-overview.

Caldwell, K., Harrison, M., Adams, M., and Triplett, N. (2009). Effect of Pilates and taijiquan training on self-efficacy, sleep quality, mood, and physical performance of college students. *Journal of Bodywork and Movement Therapy, 13*, 155-163.

Centers for Disease Control and Prevention (2009). Prevalence of autism spectrum disorders—Autism and Developmental Disabilities Network, United States, 2006. *Morbidity and Mortality Weekly Report Surveillance Summary, 58*, SS-10.

Centers for Disease Control and Prevention (2011a). Autism Fact Sheet. Retrieved May 17, 2011, from http://www.cdc.gov/NCBDDD/actearly/facts.html.

Centers for Disease Control and Prevention (2011b). Facts about Autism Spectrum Disorders. Retrieved May 25, 2011, from http://www.cdc.gov/ncbddd/autism/facts.html.

Centers for Disease Control and Prevention (2011c). Asperger Syndrome Fact Sheet. Retrieved May 25, 2011, from www.cdc.gov/ncbddd/actearly/pdf/parents_pdfs/Asperger_Syndrome.pdf.

Conant, K., Morgan, A., Muzykewicz, D., Clark, D., and Thiele, E. (2008). A karate program for improving self-concept and quality of life in childhood epilepsy: Results of a pilot study. *Epilepsy Behavior, 12*(1), 61-65.

Daniels, K., and Thornton, E. (1992). Length of training, hostility and the martial arts: A comparison with other sporting groups. *British Journal of Sports Medicine, 26*(3), 118-120.

Gleser, J., Margulies, J., Nyaka, M., Porat, B., Mendelberg, B., and Wertman, E. (1992). Physical and psychosocial benefits of modified judo practice for blind, mentally retard children: A pilot study. *Perceptual and Motor Skills, 74* (3 part 1), 915-925.

Kim, Y., Leventhal, B., Koh, Y., Fombonne, E., Laska, et al. (2011). Prevalence of autism spectrum disorders in a total population sample. *American Journal of Psychiatry.* Epub version published May 9, 2011, doi: 10.1176/appi.ajp.2011.10101532.

KRAMER, E. (2011). Life is growth: An adapted martial arts program. Unpublished graduate thesis, Harvard Graduate School of Education, Cambridge. Retrieved via personal e-mail May 18, 2011.

LAMARRE, B., AND NOSANCHUK, T. (1999). Judo—the gentle way: A replication of studies on martial arts and aggression. *Perceptual and Motor Skills, 88* (3 part 1), 992-996.

Lakes, K., AND Hoyt, W. (2004). Promoting self-regulation through school-based martial arts training. *Applied Developmental Psychology, 25,* 283-302.

LUNDSTRÖM, S., CHANG, Z., KEREKES, N., GUMPERT C., RÅSTAM, M., GILLBERG, C., LICHTENSTEIN, P., AND ANCKARSÄTER, H. (2011). Autistic-like traits and their association with mental health problems in two nationwide twin cohorts of children and adults. *Psychological Medicine, 22,* 1-11.

MAYO CLINIC.COM. (2011). Asperger's Syndrome. Retrieved May 17, 2011, from http://www.mayoclinic.com/health/aspergers-syndrome/DS00551.

MÜLLER, E., SCHULER, A., AND YATES, G. (2008). Social challenges and supports from the perspective of individuals with Asperger syndrome and other autism spectrum disorder. *Autism, 12*(12), 173-190.

MUKADDES, N., HERGÜNER, S., AND TANIDIR, C. (2010). Psychiatric disorders in individuals with high-functioning autism and Asperger's disorder: Similarities and differences. *World Journal of Biological Psychiatry, 11*(8), 964-971.

NATIONAL INSTITUTE OF NEUROLOGICAL DISORDERS AND STROKE. NINDS pervasive developmental disorders information page. Retrieved May 9, 2011, from http://www.ninds.nih.gov/disorders/pdd/pdd.htm.

RIMMER, J., YAMAKI, K., LOWRY, B., WANG, E., AND VOGEL, L. (2010). Obesity and obesity-related secondary conditions in adolescents with intellectual/developmental disabilities. *Journal of Intellectual Disability Research, 54,* 787-794.

SEBASTIAN, C., BLAKEMORE, S., AND CHARMAN, T. (2009) Reactions to ostracism in adolescents with autism spectrum conditions. *Journal of Autism and Developmental Disorders, 39,* 1122-1130.

SHIFFLETT, C. (2000). *Aikido: Exercises for teaching and training.* Sewickley, PA: Round Earth Publishing.

TWYMAN, K., SAYLOR C., SAIA, D., MAIAS, M., TAYLOR, L., AND SPRATT, E. (2010). Bullying and ostracism experiences in children with special health care needs. *Journal of Developmental and Behavioral Pediatrics, 31*(1), 1-8.

VICKERSTAFF, S., HERIOT, S., WONG, M., LOPES, A., AND DOSSETOR, D. (2007). Intellectual ability, self-perceived social competence, and depressive symptomatology in children with high-functioning autistic spectrum disorders. *Journal of Autism and Developmental Disorders, 37*(9), 1647-1664.

WALL, R. (2005). Tai Chi and mindfulness-based stress reduction in a Boston Public Middle School. *Journal of Pediatric Health Care, 1*(4), 230-237.

WOODWARD, T. (2009). A review of the effects of martial arts practice on health. *Wisconsin Medical Journal, 108*(1), 40-43.

WRIGHT, P., WHITE, K., AND GAEBLER-SPIRA, D. (2004). Exploring the relevance of the personal and social responsibility model in adapted physical activity: A collective case study. *Journal of Teaching in Physical Education, 23*(1), 71-87.

ZIVIN, G., HASSAN, N., DEPAULA G., MONTI, D., HARLAN, C., HOSSAIN, K., AND PATTERSON, K. (2001). An effective approach to violence prevention: Traditional martial arts in middle school. *Adolescence,* 36 (fall), 443-459.

INDEX

academic performance, 2, 4, 7, 9, 11, 18-19
acquired behavior, 54, 57, 87
aggression, 10, 51-61, 66, 69-70, 81, 85-87, 99, 104
aikido, 99-100, 102-110
anger, 31, 41, 52-53
asperger syndrome, 70, 101
Attention-deficit Disorder, 65-68, 75
Autism Spectrum Disorders, 99-104, 109-110
awareness, 2, 7, 24, 31-32, 42, 44, 100, 102-104, 109
belt rank, 1, 5, 7-9, 13-14, 60, 82, 86-87
Buddhism, 2, 35, 45-46, 48, 83
bullying, 24, 29-30, 49
character building, 81, 83-85
commitment, 6-7,
competition, 74, 83-84, 87
confidentiality, 66, 71-72, 75
conflict, 21-26, 28-29, 31, 33-38, 48-50, 82
desire to learn, 39-40
discipline, 59-60, 62, 81, 84-85, 87-88
doctor visits, 4, 7-8, 13-14, 16
empty self, 22
enrollment, 1-6, 11-13, 15, 17-18, 58, 65, 87, 100, 103
expectations, 11-13, 15, 17-18
fear of injury, 24, 52, 72
fight-or-flight response, 26, 28, 31, 33, 49
frustration, 53-54
Funakoshi, Gichin, 22-23, 35, 60
gender, 1, 5-6, 9, 12, 101
hyperactivity disorder, 65-67, 69-70, 75
imitation, 54-56, 59, 61

instructors of martial arts, 1, 6, 11, 21, 24, 29, 36-37, 39-40, 46, 51, 59-60, 61-62, 65-67, 70-76, 80, 82, 100, 103, 110
juvenile delinquency, 36, 60-61, 81, 85-87
karate, 1-19, 21-22, 35-36, 60, 62
ki exercises, 104-109
kick-boxing, 2
length of training, 8, 86
Martial Arts for Peace, 21-22, 29, 31, 34, 36-37
mental conditioning, 22-23, 25-29, 31-33, 38, 50, 54
mental health, 2, 4-5, 10, 30, 32-33, 36, 45, 48-49, 83, 87, 94, 99, 101, 103
Min, Ken, 80
model of behavior, 51, 54-55, 57-62, 74
nature environment, 41
non-violence, 24, 83
observation, 1-2, 31-32, 51, 54-56, 58, 74, 101
ostracism, 102
peer presure, 10
physical coordination, 2, 9, 102, 104, 109
physical health, 1, 4, 7-8, 13-14, 16, 45, 50, 102
physical improvement, 4, 7, 11-17, 18, 61
resocialization, 9
respect, 10, 38, 59, 62, 81-82, 89, 91-92
role playing, 21, 29, 49
school attendance, 4, 7-8, 13-14, 16
school teachers, 70
self-confidence, 1-2, 4-5, 7, 9-12, 14, 16, 18, 85, 87

self-discipline, 4-5, 7, 9, 11-12, 14, 16, 18, 81
self-defense, 4, 6, 9, 11-13, 15, 17-18, 21-25, 27, 35, 37, 47-49, 52, 82-83
self-esteem, 1-2, 7, 9, 71, 81, 8588, 92-93, 99, 102-103
self-regulation, 57
sensitivity, 9, 24, 75, 102
Shotokan Karate, 22
Shorinji Kempo, 44-46
shu-ha-ri concept, 25, 27, 38
social environment, 9, 54-59, 84, 100-102
moral standards, 57, 59

sport, 6, 10, 22-23, 59, 68, 80-81, 83-86, 93-94
story telling, 34
taekwondo, 68-70, 79-94
Take Nami-do, 21
teacher-student relationship, 46, 59
traditions/modern martial arts, 1-2, 9-10, 25, 59-62, 82-84, 86-87, 93-94
training, 1-4, 6, 10, 28, 32, 36, 47, 49, 60-61, 66-69, 72-76, 79-88, 91-93, 99
University of California-Berkeley, Martial Arts Program, 80
violence, 51, 53, 56, 58-60, 62, 81, 99
violence in the media, 55-56, 58

Printed in Great Britain
by Amazon